Psychopathology and Function

A GUIDE FOR OCCUPATIONAL THERAPISTS

BETTE R. BONDER, PhD, OTR

Gary Kielhofner, Editor
MENTAL HEALTH PROFESSIONAL SERIES

SLACK Incorporated, 6900 Grove Road, Thorofare, New Jersey 08086

Editorial Director: Cheryl D. Willoughby
Publisher: Harry C. Benson

Printed in the United States of America

Library of Congress Catalog Card Number: 88-43158

ISBN: 1-55642-076-5

Published by: SLACK Incorporated
               6900 Grove Road
               Thorofare, NJ 08086-9447

Last digit is print number: 10   9   8   7   6   5   4   3

Dedication

For Pat, Aaron, and Jordan

Contents

Preface

Any health care provider working in mental health recognizes the importance of psychiatric diagnosis. Many decisions in the mental health system are based on the label which the patient carries. However, most mental health professionals are also aware of the limitations of this label. Most important for occupational therapists, it provides relatively little information about what the individual needs to accomplish in order to survive, or the activities the individual wants to be able to do in order to maintain a high level of life satisfaction. In addition, it does not inform the therapist about the individual's ability to perform those activities.

While occupational therapists must function within the system, their perspective about clients may be markedly different from that of other team members. This is desirable, since optimal well-being is comprised of many factors: physical health, functional abilities, attitudes, and so on. All these must be considered in providing the most effective intervention. However, professionals must be able to communicate with each other, and for better or for worse, the diagnostic system is the way in which this communication occurs.

This text integrates the perspectives of medicine and occupational therapy, enabling the occupational therapist to convey information in ways the physician (usually a psychiatrist) and other team members will understand. It also enables the occupational therapist to interpret what team members are saying about the client in terms of the goals of therapy. While this understanding is crucial, it is also important for occupational therapists to maintain their unique perspective, and to make their vital contribution to effective intervention. It is only through this interaction of views that the best possible outcomes can be assured for the service recipient.

Acknowledgements

This project would not have been possible without the help of many individuals. The idea for the book originated with Gary Kielhofner, who has provided invaluable support and feedback throughout its development. Others who reviewed the manuscript and gave helpful suggestions include Jaimie Munoz and the occupational therapy students at the University of Illinois at Chicago.

Special thanks are due to Janet Davies, who spent hours in the library unearthing sometimes obscure references, and to Karen Bradley for preparation of the manuscript through its many revisions.

My husband, Pat Bray, and my sons, Aaron and Jordan, served as my personal cheering squad during the completion of what they labeled "the world's longest homework assignment." They have my heartfelt thanks.

Introduction

The field of mental health has undergone vast changes in the last 25 years. Experimentally validated information about both etiology and treatment of psychiatric disorders has grown enormously, allowing for increasingly effective intervention and, in many instances, more positive prognosis. New information has changed the face of mental health treatment for the individual and, at the same time, altered the systems in which intervention is offered.

In spite of the increase in knowledge, much remains to be learned. The etiology of some syndromes remains a mystery, with heated debate continuing about others as to whether they are the result of biology, environment, learning, or some combination of these. Treatment is, in some instances, still a matter of trial and error, with providers making educated guesses about which of the existing interventions which make a difference. Even when a specific therapy is generally accepted as treatment of choice, the reasons for its efficacy may be poorly understood.

At the same time, health care in general has become increasingly complex, both in terms of treatment and the systems in which care is delivered. Patients, their families and employers, third party payers and health care providers all struggle with issues about quality of care, cost, and the rights of the various interested parties. Occupational therapists, like other health care providers have had to adapt to these increasing complexities in order to continue to provide high quality care.

Occupational therapy as a profession originated in mental health (Bruce & Borg, 1987). The earliest therapists provided activities which were thought "useful" and "healthful," as "moral treatment" emerged as a theory for intervention. Meyer (1977) believed mental illness to be a "problem of living," and felt that a balance of work, leisure, and rest would restore health.

The emerging beliefs of occupational therapy fit within the two primary forms of treatment employed by physicians and other mental health care providers at that time. For individuals who were psychotic (severely disturbed and out of contact with reality), removal from the environment and placement in an institution was the norm. It was felt that these disorders were largely intractable, and little could be done except to relieve the families of the burden of caring for their bizarre relatives. There was some suspicion that these illnesses had a physical component, as a result of which insulin shock, psychosurgery, and, later, electroshock treatments were employed. For those who were "neurotic" (emotionally disturbed but in contact with reality), psychoanalysis or other verbal therapies were implemented, usually while the patient continued to reside at home. This form of treatment often meant years of intensive verbal therapy focused on discussions of experiences which might have molded maladaptive emotional reactions.

The most striking change in mental health care was the discovery of a variety of psychopharmacological agents in the middle of this century. These drugs made it possible to control many psychotic symptoms, as well as depression and anxiety. At the same time, a variety of new theories about behavior increased the range of therapies from which treatment choices were made. Behavior therapy, cognitive therapy, and family therapies are among the alternatives which have emerged. These theories have been investigated with a variety of research methodologies, so that effectiveness can be more clearly established.

Many of the new therapies are brief. As contrasted with earlier types of interventions which may have continued for years, many of the newer types of treatment are designed to reach maximum effectiveness within a few weeks or months. In addition, many are provided outside of institutional settings, in community mental health centers, day treatment centers, or other community based facilities.

In addition to (and perhaps in response to) the rapid growth of knowledge about psychiatric disorders, there has been a proliferation of mental health professions. Early in the century, psychiatrists, psychologists, social workers, and nurses were the primary providers of care. Added to the list now, in addition to occupational therapists, are vocational counselors, recreation, art, music, dance therapists and many others. The roles of these professionals may be blurred, with overlap among them. To function effectively together, each must bring a strong sense of professional identity, a clear picture of what he or she may contribute to the well being of the client.

There is now one more interested party in mental health care, the entity which funds treatment. It was not uncommon, earlier in the century, for the individual or the family to pay directly for services received. The norm now is for an employer, an insurance company, or the government to support care. As costs have soared, these organizations have become increasingly involved in decision making about the kinds of care to be provided, the circumstances under which they will be provided, and the duration. There is constant review of the efficacy of treatment, and the payers demand that the effectiveness of each intervention be demonstrated by observable changes in behavior or symptoms.

All these factors have made service provision in mental health a complex proposition. The well-being of the individual is now frequently weighed against the interests of the various parties involved in each situation. It is in this complex system that occupational therapists must now operate, must strive to provide quality services to individuals and families with mental health problems.

In order to function effectively, occupational therapists must have a clear understanding of the needs of the individual, of the system in which they are providing care, of the roles of other professionals, and of their own contributions to care. There are several factors which must be considered. First, when occupational therapists offer treatment in mental health, they generally do so as part of a treatment team. This team is usually headed by a psychiatrist, a physician with specialized training in mental illness. The medical background of the team leader is significant, because it contributes to the importance of diagnosis as a starting place for treatment. While this delineation of authority is less prominent in some types of community treatment environments, diagnosis may still be emphasized.

As noted above, payment for services is almost always provided, at least in part, by someone other than the identified patient. In most cases, the other is an insurance company or the government. Increasingly, employers are providing their own insurance for employees, and are acting as the third party payers. As these others pay, they are involved in decisions about care. Their interests may be somewhat different than those of the patient, with cost containment an important factor. They are interested in service which is effective, but is within reasonable cost limits. One of the ways in which they control costs is by reviewing diagnoses and prognoses and paying only for treatments which have been demonstrated through research and practice to be effective for the specific disorder. Thus diagnosis assumes importance in terms of the kinds of treatment which are likely to be reimbursed.

In focusing on the individual's ability to perform those tasks required in daily life, occupational therapists respond to both the needs of the patient and the wishes of third party payers. Enhancing function may serve to make individuals less dependent, enable them to live without support from the environment, or minimize the need for such support. Thus occupational therapists provide a vital service with the potential to increase function and quality of life and decrease costs.

However, occupational therapists must work within the existing treatment milieu. This presents several difficulties. First, and most importantly, psychiatric diagnosis does not always predict functional performance. As Williams (1988) indicates "(diagnosis) does not imply that all people with a particular mental disorder are alike; on the contrary they may differ in many important ways that can affect treatment and outcome" (p.203). Individuals labeled as schizophrenic may function in very different ways, some able to live reasonably independently, others almost totally dependent. Second, it may be difficult for occupational therapists to articulate their goals in a system where diagnosis and symptoms generally reflect psychological rather than functional characteristics. For example, schizophrenics may be described in terms of cognitive and sensory distortions, rather than in terms of the ways in which those distortions affect their ability to work or care for themselves.

The purpose of this book is to describe for therapists the diagnostic system currently used in the United States and to discuss the role of occupational therapy within that system. The emergence of the current classification system, the Diagnostic and Statistical Manual III-Revised (DSM-III-R) (American Psychiatric Association, 1987), will be reviewed. The relationship of psychiatric treatment to the occupational therapy process will be considered. Then, the DSM-III-R categories will be described with regard to incidence of the disorder, symptomatology, etiology, and prognosis. Most important, functional performance will be examined for the various categories, both in terms of skills (motor, cognitive, sensory, etc.), and activities (work, leisure, activities of daily living, etc.). Discussion of the implications of performance for occupational therapy intervention will be included. The final chapter deals with psychotropic medications. Medication has emerged as a primary form of treatment by psychiatrists, regardless of orientation. All mental health professionals should understand the effects of these agents as well as the potential side-effects. Occupational therapy treatment must often be planned with these effects in mind. For this reason, medication as a form of intervention will be considered in some detail.

By developing a clear understanding of psychopathology and psychiatric diagnosis, and the role of occupational therapy within that context, occupational therapists can be best equipped to provide optimal service to clients.

References

American Psychiatric Association, Task Force on Nomenclature, (1987). *Diagnostic and Statistical Manual of Mental Disorders* (3rd ed. revised). Washington, DC: American Psychiatric Association.

Bruce, M.A., & Borg, B.(1987). *Frames of Reference in Psychosocial Occupational Therapy.* Thorofare, NJ: Slack.

Meyer, A. (1977). The philosophy of occupation therapy. *American Journal of Occupational Therapy, 31,* 639-642.

Williams, J.B.W. (1988) Psychiatric classification. In J.A. Talbott, R.E. Hales, & S.C. Yudofsky (Eds.) *The American Psychiatric Press Textbook of Psychiatry.* Washington, D.C.: American Psychiatric Press, p. 201-223.

Chapter 1
Psychiatric Diagnosis and the Classification System

There are a large number of theories about psychiatric disorders with widely varying implications for intervention, including behavioral, analytic, and biomedical. This creates a dilemma for providers. Without a common ground for understanding, communication among professionals becomes impossible. The resolution of the dilemma has been the development of a common system of classification, the *Diagnostic and Statistical Manual (DSM)*. Since its appearance in 1952, it has undergone several revisions, with the current edition known as the *Diagnostic and Statistical Manual III-Revised (DSM-III-R, 1987)*. It is through the *DSM-III-R* that mental health professionals can converse regardless of theoretical orientation. As has been noted, "mental health professionals need a common language with which to communicate about the types of psychological problems for which they assume professional responsibility. A diagnosis is simply a way of summarizing a large amount of information into a shorthand term" (Spitzer, Skodal, Gibbon, & Williams, 1983, p. xvi).

Communication is a vital function of a classification system, but there are others. According to Williams (1988), such a system provides a guide to cause, and by extension, assessment and treatment of disorders. For example, "physical" disorders must be distinguished from psychiatric syndromes as treatment clearly revolves around such distinctions (Hall, Gardner, Stickney, LeCann, & Popkin, 1980). In addition, description of the known characteristics of each disorder is vital to efforts to improve diagnostic reliability and the ability to discriminate among disorders. Finally, classification assists in research to further examine causes of mental disturbance and treatment. Without a shared system for identification of distinguishable disorders, such research becomes almost impossible. For example, diagnostic criteria assist in identifying specific groups of individuals to be studied, behaviors to be examined, and outcomes that are of interest to the researcher.

Emergence of the DSM

In 1840, the United States had a one-category classification system for mental illness, that category being "Idiocy" (Williams, 1988). By 1880, the system had increased to eight categories. Over time, as understanding and awareness increased, the classification system was refined, eventually being formalized as a chapter in the *International Classification of Diseases (ICD)*, now in its ninth edition (World Health Organization, 1979), and as the *DSM*.

The *Diagnostic and Statistical Manual, Mental Disorders*, later to be known as *DSM-I*, was published in 1952 by the American Psychiatric Association (APA). It was a major breakthrough for the field of mental health, as it provided the first comprehensive volume describing the range of mental disorders. The descriptions were quite general, however, making diagnosis unreliable. As psychiatric knowledge grew, it became clear that a revision was needed.

DSM-II appeared in 1968, following 3 years of work by the APA. It coincided with the eighth revision of the *ICD*. The differences between *DSM-I* and *DSM-II* were minor, with some changes in the names of syndromes and minor changes in descriptive language. Like *DSM-I*, though, descriptions were general and often vague. A major criticism of both *DSM-I* and *DSM-II* was the poor reliability of diagnosis. This means that professionals were often unable to consistently identify the same disorder in a specific patient (Klerman, 1988), or that a diagnosis might be changed over time even if nothing had happened to change the behavior or symptoms of the individual.

DSM-III represented a major change in the nature of the diagnostic process. As with *DSM-II*, its development coincided with a revision of the *ICD*. American psychiatrists were concerned that the *ICD-9* lacked many specific diagnoses that were well-accepted in the United States on the basis of research data. There was also concern that the glossary was inadequate in the area of mental health (Williams, 1988).

Furthermore, in the 1960s and 1970s, there was heated debate about the nature and even existence of mental illness. Szasz (1974), for example, argued that mental illness was a cultural phenomenon, rather than any sort of disease entity. He suggested that mental illness was used as a label to explain deviant, and therefore socially unacceptable, behavior, and that the purpose of the label was to provide an excuse to control such behavior. Supporting this argument was the poor reliability of diagnoses. If two professionals were unlikely to make the same diagnosis of a patient, Szasz argued, perhaps it was because they were responding to cultural imperatives rather than to any real problem with the individual's behavior.

The 1970s saw several advances that contributed to the discussion. Foremost among these was the vastly increased knowledge about psychopharmacology and biology. For the first time, biological factors in mental disturbance could be identified, both in terms of genetic and biochemical characteristics. At the same time, research capabilities were enhanced through development of new research methodologies and through development of reliable clinical instruments (Klerman, 1988); ie, that professionals became consistent in their views of specific patients, and diagnosis was stable over time if the patient did not change. Among the categorizations developed during that period were the *Research Diagnostic Criteria (RDC)* (Spitzer, Forman and Nee, 1979). The emergence of such measures demonstrated that it was possible to provide clear, consistent guidelines that allowed for discrimination among diagnostic categories.

Thus, in 1974, the APA appointed a committee to begin development of *DSM-III,* a task that ultimately took 6 years. Both the process of development and the ultimate product were novel, representing a significant departure from DSM-II. The process involved not only a great deal of committee work to develop descriptions and diagnostic criteria, but also a major research effort to validate diagnoses and determine reliability in a systematic fashion. During the research phase, more than 12,000 individuals were evaluated (Spitzer, Forman and Nee, 1979). Clinicians from around the United States completed reports and commented on any difficulties using the system.

The inter-rater reliability studies involved 796 patients, each of whom was evaluated by two clinicians. Because these were field studies, some variables were poorly controlled, but even so, the new classification system was demonstrated to have reliability coefficients in the range of .7 (Axis I) to .6 (Axis II) (Williams, 1985), meaning, roughly, that professionals agreed 60% to 70% of the time. The attempt to confirm reliability was, itself, novel. It should be noted that some later studies have found lower reliability, especially for Axis II (Mellsop, Varhgese, Joshua, & Hicks, 1982).

The product was notably different from *DSM-II.* First, the number of diagnoses was expanded to more than 150. In addition, descriptions were designed to be as specific as possible, with criteria about constellations of symptoms, onset of the disorder, and duration and probable course. This specificity was an important factor in assuring reliability and represented the first classification to provide operational criteria (Klerman, 1988). Operational criteria are specific, observable characteristics that describe a particular syndrome or disorder. It is also noteworthy that it provided descriptive psychopathology rather than inferred etiology. In other words, the guide described what the clinician saw, not what caused it. In addition, descriptions were largely atheoretical, that is, without reference to particular theories or points of view, making the product an effective mechanism for communication among therapists subscribing to divergent treatment philosophies (Williams, 1988).

In addition, *DSM-III* acknowledged that diagnosis alone might not provide sufficient data to implement treatment. As a result, several new categories were developed to provide additional information, making it the first multiaxial classification system (Klerman, 1988). These axes made it possible not only to name a syndrome, but also to identify the type of personality of the individual in whom the problem was occurring; accompanying significant medical conditions to treatment and prognosis; levels of stress encountered by the individual; and recent levels of function.

Inclusion of this last axis is of particular importance to occupational therapists, as it represents an acknowledgment that diagnosis alone does not adequately describe function. It is also noteworthy that Axis V appears to be the most reliable of the axes with an r somewhere between .7 and .8 (Williams, 1988). Simply put, this means that there is agreement among raters 70% to 80% of the time.

In *DSM-III*, categories were hierarchical, based on the assumption that disorders higher on the hierarchy had symptoms found in those lower, but not the opposite. Later research has questioned this assumption (Boyd, Burke, Gruenberg, Holzer, Rae, 1984), and this was one of the many findings that led to the almost immediate effort to revise the *DSM-III*. *DSM-III-R* was published in 1987 and reflects advances in scientific knowledge. One change, for example, was the omission of the assumption of heirarchies (Williams, 1988). Although the changes were minor, they reflect an effort to resolve problems with *DSM-III* and an effort to disseminate new knowledge as quickly as possible.

Not all the development of the classification systems was done on the basis of scientific evidence. Klerman (1988) notes that politics affected several of the categories, and, as work begins for the projected publication of *DSM-IV* in 1992, political arguments rage while scientific work continues. One dispute, for example, relates to the inclusion of a diagnosis of "self-defeating personality." Feminists argued that this validated the tendency of the legal system to "blame the victim" for crimes committed against him or her (for example, that battered wives bring the problem on themselves). This particular dispute was temporarily resolved by the inclusion in *DSM-III-R* of an appendix that listed potential diagnoses needing further study and verification. Another dispute was based in theory. *DSM-III-R* purports to be atheoretical, but this led to the omission of constructs deemed important by one group or another. Psychoanalysts and other dynamically oriented therapists, for example, wanted to see defense mechanisms added as a sixth axis (Frances & Cooper, 1981). This conflict was resolved by the inclusion of these terms in an extensive glossary. Analysts were further dismayed by the deletion of any category called neurosis. Their argument that this omission in itself constituted a theoretical statement was countered by the assertion that "neurosis" specifies intrapsychic conflict as an etiology (Bayer & Spitzer, 1985). This dispute is as yet unresolved.

Other substantive concerns have been raised. Treece (1982) suggested that substance abuse is so pervasive that these disorders should have an axis of their own. Fleck (1983) expressed concern that family factors were not adequately represented in the five axis framework, making diagnosis difficult for family therapists. Several individuals have suggested that both stressors and function should be separated on the basis of social and vocational factors, either as 2 x 2 tables within the existing axes or as separate axes (Linn & Spitzer, 1982). This argument holds that social and vocational function may be quite different for given individuals, and that provision of only one axis to summarize these performance areas often leads to an inaccurate picture of the individual's capabilities. Thus, the development of the classification system can be seen as a complex scientific and political process, which has involved physicians, psychologists, social workers, and some political or special interest groups. In spite of, or perhaps because of, the conflict that surrounds development, each revision has represented an improvement both in format and content, and there is reason to believe that DSM-IV will follow this trend.

Format of DSM-III-R

As noted, *DSM-III-R* is a multiaxial classification system comprised of five axes. Axis I represents psychiatric diagnosis; Axis II, personality disorders; Axis III, significant accompanying medical conditions; Axis IV, degree of stress within the 12 months preceding diagnosis; and Axis V, level of function. On this last axis, two numbers are listed: current level of function and highest level of function within the past 12 months. Diagnosis on all five axes is designed to provide maximal information about the individual's condition. (See Fig. 1-1)

Figure 1-1
DSM-III-R Axes

Axis I	Clinical Symptoms V Codes
Axis II	Developmental Disorders Personality Disorders
Axis III	Physical Disorders and Conditions

Figure 1-1 *continued*

Axis IV	Severity of Psychosocial Stressors
Axis V	Global Assessment of Function

Appendix A contains the summary pages from *DSM-III-R*. The categories listed there are discussed in detail in the body of the text, with clarifying examples of behavior, and specific symptoms that must be present to support a given diagnosis. This description includes considerations such as duration of symptoms and course of the disorder.

Axis I includes diagnoses of specific psychiatric syndromes or disorders. Earlier classifications were divided into psychotic and neurotic categories, psychotic disorders being largely those for which some biological etiology was known or presumed, whereas neurotic disorders were those for which etiology was unclear (Klerman, 1988). Increasing numbers of disorders have been demonstrated to have some biological component, making this distinction less valid. Thus, it does not appear in *DSM-III* or *DSM-III-R*, and the term neurosis has been dropped.

Each *DSM-III-R* diagnostic category includes a description of major features of the disorder, the symptoms that must be present to warrant the diagnosis, and a discussion of accompanying features that may or may not be present. Age of onset and course of the disorder are described, as are predisposing factors, prevalence, and familial pattern. A section on impairment briefly discusses the social and vocational implications of the disorder. Complications that may occur are included and, finally, a discussion of differential diagnosis provides a summary of the characteristics that distinguish the disorder from others and a list of other diagnoses to consider if criteria do not fit the presenting picture.

Axis II lists personality and developmental disorders, which are defined as long-standing patterns of adaptation. Individuals may have psychiatric diagnoses without personality disorders, or vice versa, but they often accompany each other. A distinguishing characteristic of a personality disorder is its usually negative effect on those around the individual (Klerman, 1988), frequently resulting in a disordered social system. Developmental disorders are included on this axis, as they are viewed as having long term consequences for adaptation.

Axis III allows for diagnosis of coexisting medical conditions, coded according to the *ICD-9* categories. Medical conditions that might affect the course of the psychiatric disorder or the types of treatments to be implemented are noted on this axis, as are those that might have an impact on overall function.

Axis IV describes psychosocial stressors. Both severity and duration of the stressors are noted. As will be seen in later chapters, presence or absence of these stress factors may affect the development of a psychiatric problem, and almost certainly influences the outcome of treatment (Paykel, 1978). It should be noted that different stressors are identified for adults and for children and adolescents.

Axis V reflects the individual's highest level of function within the 12 months preceding diagnosis, as well as current level of function. Psychological, social, and vocational functioning are rated on a 0 to 90 point scale, with general descriptions of each 10 point range to provide guidance in making an assessment. This is, at present, the most subjective of the axes as specific behaviors are not included. However, a moderate correlation has been noted between severity of symptoms and function (Klerman, 1988), i.e. there is a moderate relationship between the degree of psychological impairment and performance. This axis was included in an attempt to acknowledge strengths of the client as well as deficits (thus highest level of function rather than average level of function). A moderate negative correlation has been found between Axes IV and V (Klerman, 1988), meaning that stress is inversely related to function. In spite of its relative subjectivity, this is, as has been mentioned, the most reliable of the axes (Axis III has not been subjected to any reliability studies). Appendix A provides a complete outline of the *DSM-III-R* categories, with reference to the pages in *DSM-III-R* where expanded discussion of each diagnosis can be found.

Figure 1-2 provides the description of one common diagnosis, dysthymia, as it appeared in *DSM-I*, *DSM-II*, *DSM-III*, and now as it is seen in *DSM-III-R*. Among the obvious differences is the change in name from depressive neurosis. Increasing specificity can be noted in each revision, increasing the probability of reliable diagnosis and thus the clarity of therapeutic choice. (See Fig. 1-2, pp. 8-11.)

What follows in this text is discussion of the relationship of diagnosis to occupational therapy and consideration of each major diagnostic category with emphasis on what is known or theorized about etiology and course of the disorders, the types of treatments currently being employed, and the efficacy of those treatments. Most importantly, that information will be linked to probable effects on the occupational performance of the individual, and recommendations made about potential interventions for occupational therapy.

Figure 1-2

Changes in the Diagnosis
of Depression DSM-I to DSM-III-R

DSM-I (1952)	000-x06 Depressive reaction
	The anxiety in this reaction is allayed, and hence partially relieved, by depression and self-depreciation. The reaction is precipitated by a current situation, frequently by some loss sustained by the patient, and is often associated with a feeling of guilt for past failures or deeds. The degree of the reaction in such cases is dependent upon the intensity of the patient's ambivalent feeling toward his loss (love, possession) as well as upon the realistic circumstances of the loss. The term is synonymous with "reactive depression" and is to be differentiated from the corresponding psychotic reaction. In this differentiation, points to be considered are (1) life history of patient, with special reference to mood swings (suggestive of psychotic reaction), to the personality structure (neurotic or cyclothymic) and to precipitating environmental factors and (2) absence of malignant symptoms (hypochondriacal preoccupation, agitation, delusions, particularly somatic, hallucinations, severe guilt feelings, intractable insomnia, suicidal ruminations, severe psychomotor retardation, profound retardation of thought, stupor).
DSM-II (1968)	300.4 Depressive neurosis
	This disorder is manifested by an excessive reaction of depression due to an internal conflict or to an identifiable event such as the loss of a love object or cherished possession. It is to be distinguished from Involutional melancholia (q.v.) and Manic-depressive illness (q.v.) Reactive depressions or Depressive reactions are to be classified here.
DSM-III (1980)	Diagnostic criteria for Dysthymic Disorder
	A. During the past two years (or one year for children and adolescents) the individual has been bothered most or all of the time by symptoms characteristic of the depressive syndrome but that are not of sufficient severity and duration to meet the criteria for a major depressive episode (although a major depressive episode may be superimposed on Dysthymic Disorder). B. The manifestations of the depressive syndrome may be relatively persistent or separated by periods of normal mood lasting a few days to a few weeks, but no more that a few months at a time. C. During the depressive periods there is either prominent depressed mood (e.g., sad, blue, down in the dumps, low) or

Figure 1-2 *continued*

DSM-III (1980)	Diagnostic criteria for Dysthymic Disorder
	marked loss of interest or pleasure in all, or almost all, usual activities and pastimes. D. During the depressive period at least three of the following symptoms are present: (1) insomnia or hypersomnia (2) low energy level or chronic tiredness (3) feelings of inadequacy, loss of self-esteem, or self-deprecation (4) decreased effectiveness or productivity at school, work, or home (5) decreased attention, concentration, or ability to think clearly (6) social withdrawal (7) loss of interest in or enjoyment of pleasurable activities (8) irritability or excessive anger (in children, expressed toward parents or caretakers) (9) inability to respond with apparent pleasure to praise or rewards (10) less active or talkative than usual, or feels slowed down or restless (11) pessimistic attitude toward the future, brooding about past events, or feeling sorry for self (12) tearfulness or crying (13) recurrent thoughts of death or suicide E. Absence of psychotic features, such as delusions, hallucinations, or incoherence, or loosening of associations. F. If the disturbance is superimposed on a preexisting mental disorder, such as Obsessive Compulsive Disorder or Alcohol Dependence, the depressed mood, by virtue of its intensity or effect on functioning, can be clearly distinguished from the individual's usual mood.
DSM-III-R (1987)	Diagnostic criteria for 100.40 Dysthymia
	A. Depressed mood (or can be irritable mood in children and adolescents) for most of the day, more days than not, as indicated either by subjective account or observation by others, for at least two years (one year for children and adolescents) B. Presence, while depressed, of at least two of the following:

Figure 1-2 *continued*

DSM-III-R (1987)	Diagnostic criteria for 100.40 Dysthymia
	1. poor appetite or overeating 2. insomnia or hypersomnia 3. low energy or fatigue 4. low self-esteem 5. poor concentration or difficulty making decisions 6. feelings of hopelessness C. During a two-year period (one-year for children and adolescents) of the disturbance, never without the symptoms in A for more than two months at a time. D. No evidence of an unequivocal Major Depressive Episode during the first two years (one year for children and adolescents) of the disturbance. **Note:** There may have been a previous Major Depressive Episode, provided there was a full remission (no significant signs or symptoms for six months) before development of the Dysthymia. In addition, after these two years (one year in children or adolescents) of Dysthymia, there may be superimposed episodes of Major Depression, in which case both diagnoses are given. E. Has never had a Manic Episode (p.217) or an unequivocal Hypomanic Episode (see p. 217). F. Not superimposed on a chronic psychotic disorder, such as Schizophrenia or Delusional Disorder. G. It cannot be established that an organic factor initiated and maintained the disturbance, e.g., prolonged administration of an antihypertensive medication. **Specify primary or secondary type:** **Primary type:** the mood disturbance is not related to a preexisting, chronic, nonmood, Axis I or Axis III disorder, e.g., Dependence Disorder, an Anxiety Disorder, or rheumatoid arthritis. **Secondary type:** the mood disturbance is apparently related to a preexisting, chronic, nonmood Axis I or Axis III disorder.

Figure 1-2 *continued*

DSM-III-R (1987)	Diagnostic criteria for 100.40 Dysthymia
	Specify early onset or late onset: **Early onset:** onset of the disturbance before age 21. **Late onset:** onset of the disturbance at age 21 or later.

American Psychiatric Association. Reprinted with Permission.

References

American Psychiatric Association, Task Force on Nomenclature. (1952). *Diagnostic and Statistical Manual of Mental Disorders* 1st ed. Washington, DC: American Psychiatric Association.

American Psychiatric Association, Task Force on Nomenclature. (1968). *Diagnostic and Statistical Manual of Mental Disorders* 2nd ed. Washington, DC: American Psychiatric Association.

American Psychiatric Association, Task Force on Nomenclature (1980). *Diagnostic and Statistical Manual of Mental Disorders* 3rd ed. Washington, DC: American Psychiatric Association.

American Psychiatric Association, Task Force on Nomenclature. (1987). *Diagnostic and Statistical Manual of Mental Disorders* 3rd ed., revised. Washington, DC: American Psychiatric Association.

Bayer, R. & Spitzer, R.L. (1985). Neurosis, psychodynamics, and *DSM-III*. *Archives of General Psychiatry, 42,* 187-196.

Boyd, J.H., Burke, J.D., Gruenberg, E., Holzer, C.E., & Rae, D.S. (1984). Exclusion criteria of *DSM-III*: A study of co-occurrence of heirarchy-free syndromes. *Archives of General Psychiatry, 41,* 983-989.

Fleck, S. (1983). A holistic approach to family typology and the axes of *DSM-III*. *Archives of General Psychiatry, 40,* 901-906.

Frances, A. & Cooper, A.M. (1981). Descriptive and dynamic psychiatry: A perspective on *DSM-III*. *American Journal of Psychiatry, 138,* 1198-1202.

Hall, R.C.W., Gardner, E.R., Stickney, S.K., LeCann, A.G., & Popkin, M.K. (1980). Physical illness manifesting as psychiatric disease. *Archives of General Psychiatry, 37,* 989-995.

Klerman, G.L. (1988). Classification and *DSM-III-R*. In A.M. Nicholi (Ed.),*The New Harvard Guide to Psychiatry*. Cambridge, MA:

Linn, L. & Spitzer, R.L. (1982). Implications for liason psychiatry and psychosomatic medicine. *Journal of the American Medical Association, 247,* 3207-3209.

Mellsop, G., Varghese, F., Joshua, S., & Hicks, A. (1982). The reliability of Axis II of *DSM-III*. *American Journal of Psychiatry, 139,* 1360-1361.

Paykel, E.S. (1978). Contribution of life events to causation of psychiatric illness. *Psychological Medicine, 8,* 245-253.

Spitzer, R.L., Skodol, A.E., Gibbon, M., & Williams, J.B.W. (1983). *Psychopathology: A Case Book.* New York: McGraw-Hill.

Spitzer, R.L., Forman, J.B.W., & Nee, J. (1979). *DSM-III* field trials. I: Initial interrater diagnostic reliability. *American Journal of Psychiatry, 136,* 818-820.

Szasz, T. (1974). *The Myth of Mental Illness,* 2nd ed. New York: Harper & Row.

Treece, C. (1982). *DSM-III* as a research tool. *American Journal of Psychiatry, 139,* 577-583.

World Health Organization. (1979). *International Classification of Diseases* 9th ed.*(ICD-9).* Geneva: author.

Williams, J.B.W. (1988) Psychiatric classification. In *The American Psychiatric Press Textbook of Psychiatry.* Washington, D.D.: American Psychiatric Association.

Williams, J.B.W. (1985). The multiaxial system of *DSM-III*: Where did it come from and where should it go? Archives of General Psychiatry, *42,* 181-186.

Chapter 2
DSM-III-R and Occupational Therapy

Before proceeding to a discussion of the various diagnostic categories, it is important to consider the relationship of psychiatric diagnosis to the occupational therapy process. Occupational therapists work within a system in which diagnosis is important, but their view of disorder is notably different. The difference revolves around the importance of function, the causes of dysfunction, goals of treatment, and methods for intervention. This chapter provides only a general overview, and readers should refer to texts that deal with the occupational therapy process in mental health. However, to understand how occupational therapy fits into the mental health system, some discussion of the differing views of dysfunction must be reviewed.

It is important to recognize that what constitutes psychiatric disturbance is not fixed or absolute. Porter (1987) has noted that "what is mental and what is physical, what is mad and what is bad, are not fixed points but culture relative" (p.10). Ideas have changed through the centuries about what constitutes mental illness and what interventions are appropriate. Shifts from acceptance of deviant behavior in the community to institutionalization, from rational to moral to medical treatment, from optimism to pessimism about the probability that individuals can "get better" have all been influenced by and have influenced ideas about the origins and treatments of mental disorders. Some theorists have speculated that deviance emerges from early childhood experiences (the analytic view), whereas others suspect that the problem is faulty learning (behaviorists), or a skewed set of interpretations about events (cognitive therapist). Szasz (1974) felt that psychiatric disorder did not exist, but was instead a reflection of lack of acceptance of behavior that was outside the norm.

DSM-III-R purports to be atheoretical, to apply regardless of one's view of the origins of psychiatric disturbance. However, the diagnostic process in itself reflects the medical model. It implies that there are specific syndromes or disorders that constitute discrete and distinguishable entities identified on the basis of constellations of symptoms, including psychological characteristics, behaviors, and physical findings. Thus, the model can be thought of as a disease model (Rogers, 1982). The purpose of intervention in this model is to cure disease.

It has been recognized for years that this model presents certain problems in psychiatric practice (Antonosky, 1972). Not all psychological theories fit neatly into the medical model. For example, behaviorists attempt to remediate problematic behaviors and cognitive therapists attempt to alter the ways in which clients view the world and their own situations. Neither of these approaches focuses on curing disease. Even so, the importance of the medical model to psychiatry continues to be evident in the centrality of the diagnostic process.   There are a number of reasons why diagnosis may be so important. Several of these have been noted in the previous chapter. Communication among professionals is facilitated by the common language provided by diagnosis (Spitzer, Skodal, Gibbon, & Williams, 1988). Decisions of third party payers are simplified by the process of attaching a label to a set of symptoms. It is, therefore, unlikely that the diagnostic system will disappear any time in the near future.

Psychiatrists have acknowledged that diagnosis is only loosely related to function. It was for this reason that Axis V was developed. It is clear that Axis V correlates with *severity* of disorder, rather than with specific diagnosis (Klerman, 1988).   Individuals who are diagnosed as schizophrenic may present with widely varying functional abilities: some are able to hold jobs, for instance, whereas others may require the constant attention of an inpatient psychiatric facility.

Occupational therapists focus on function, both in explaining psychiatric disorder and in intervening (Rogers, 1982). While physicians, psychiatrists in this case, focus on disease, occupational therapists focus on performance. It is quite possible to have a disease that results in no functional deficit, or at least not one that requires intervention. An individual who has a head cold has a disease, but may carry on with normal activities.

On the other hand, some individuals who have no diagnoseable disease, either physical or psychological, have deficits in performance. Children from socioeconomically deprived backgrounds may have difficulty adapting to the expectations in a school setting; adults from isolated rural settings might show performance deficits when they move to the city to take factory jobs. These do not constitute diseases in the medical sense, but occupational therapists would be concerned about remediating the performance deficits.

This view of the individual is a consistent tenet of occupational therapy regardless of the theoretical orientation of the individual. Thus, individuals who adhere to Kielhofner's (1985) Model of Human Occupation, a general systems model, and Allen's (1985) cognitive approach, a neurobiological model, would focus on function as the central concern of assessment and intervention. The specific problems identified on the basis of these theories would differ, as would the interventions, but the long term goal is to enhance function.

This perspective is reflected in the Uniform Terminology Checklist (AOTA, 1989). This is a summary of the skills and performance, which are the focus of occupational therapy (see Appendix B). Major performance areas, activities of daily living, work, and play or leisure, have been identified. For successful performance in each of these areas, a wide range of skills is needed. These include sensorimotor, cognitive, and psychosocial skills. These performance areas and skills are the focus of occupational therapy.

Reed and Sanderson (1980) list the following as the goals of occupational therapy:

1. Evaluate human behavior and function in terms of occupational performance, the components of that performance, and the required adaptive behavior.
2. Support the optimum health of each person based on the individual's needs and the community demands for occupational performance.
3. Develop, improve, re-establish, promote, or maintain normal occupational function and performance throughout the human life span.
4. Prevent, remediate, or minimize dysfunctional occupational performance and maladaptive behavior throughout the human life span (p. 11-12).

Thus, the occupational therapist examines the abilities of the individual in the identified performance areas, considers which skills are deficient and prevent maximum performance, and sets about remediating those deficits, or, in the case of the individual at risk, preventing them.

There are several ways in which the occupational therapist might approach these tasks. In psychiatry, intervention falls into three primary categories: enhancing skills and performance; altering attitudes about skills and performance; and altering the environment to maximize skills and performance.

The first category includes teaching and training. The occupational therapist might provide cooking classes, classes on job seeking, etc. Another approach is to provide practice. A client might be assigned a job in the clinic through which work-related skills can be learned. This category also includes interventions that remediate underlying skills. A child who is retarded might be provided with intense kinesthetic and proprioceptive input through swinging and spinning. According to sensory integration theory, this might better organize the central nervous system, thus enhancing higher level skills (Ayres, 1972). Another example, based on developmental theory, would be providing the same child with practice on lower level skills (for example, to balance on a balance beam) to assist the child in gradually achieving higher order skills in a step by step fashion (Bruce & Borg, 1987).

The second major type of intervention relates to the individual's attitudes and beliefs. Individuals who have been diagnosed with various psychiatric disorders often have inaccurate or skewed views of themselves. Inaccurate self-concept and lowered self-esteem are common among these individuals, regardless of specific diagnosis. These problems may lead to ineffective performance. Such individuals may not know that they can do particular activities, or may feel a chronic sense of failure. In some instances they may not know what they feel, or may need help expressing emotions. Providing these clients with success experiences may bolster sagging self-esteem, and review of performance on a variety of activities may allow more accurate self-assessment. The model of human occupation (Kielhofner, 1985) suggests that clients need to have and be aware of their own valued goals to perform effectively. Expressive arts, including drawing, dance, and creative writing, can facilitate expression of emotion.

The third form that intervention typically takes is environmental modification. It has been theorized that some individuals do not have great capacity to modify their own performance, but that they may benefit from modifications in the environment that reduce demand (Allen, 1985). Another way of viewing this set of interventions is that many individuals do not know how to construct for themselves the most supportive environments, and that they can benefit from learning how to do this. It seems likely that setting can influence the performance of the individual, and that modification of the setting, whether by the therapist or the individual, will maximize function (Rogers, 1983).

The primary modality employed by occupational therapists in all these areas is activity. This includes all the kinds of activities in which individuals normally engage: routine daily activities such as cooking, cleaning, and self-care; work activities, including studying; leisure and play, including sports and crafts; and expressive activities such as art, writing, and dance. The belief is that a balance of these activities promotes the best possible quality of life for the individual (Meyer, 1977). Figure 2-1 lists the primary areas of occupational therapy focus and some of the specific goals and modalities that might be used to intervene.

Thus, a psychiatrist might look at a client who presents with depressed mood and lethargy and say: "Here is someone who has a dysthymic disorder. Let us treat the client with antidepressant medication and with verbal therapy to allow him to ventilate his feelings." The occupational therapist might look at the same client and say: "Here is someone who has a pervasive sense of failure and no clear goals in life. Let us provide him with activities that will affirm his strengths and help him identify some goals which will give his life meaning." The two approaches are clearly different. In the best possible situation, they are complementary, each providing the client with something that will enhance his satisfaction with life, as well as his ability to contribute to society.

Figure 2-1
Occupational Therapy Goals and Treatments

Objective	Sample Treatment Goals	Sample Approaches
1. Enhance skills and performance	a. Improve ADL skills in: grooming, hygiene	a. Education (teach skill or performance)
	b. Improve ADL skills in: budgeting and money management, housekeeping, etc.	b. Practice (provide experience)
	c. Enhance work related skills: job seeking, interviewing, relating to co-workers	c. Reinforcement—used alone or in connection with education
	d. Improve orientation	d. Reality orientation
		e. Sensory stimulation
2. Self-image and self-expression	a. Increase self-esteem	a. Provide activities with high probability of successful outcome
	b. Encourage accurate self-assessment	b. Provide feedback on outcomes
	c. Increase ability to recognize emotions	c. Use of expressive activities: drawing, painting, writing, dance
3. Modify environment to maximize function	a. Reduce stress of environment	a. Move to smaller community, more structured living space
	b. Provide performance cues	b. Reduce clutter, label cabinets
	c. Encourage environmental support	c. Link to community services, church groups

You will note in the chapters that follow that the suggestions for occupational therapy intervention appear somewhat repetitive. This is because the book is organized around psychiatric symptoms rather than symptoms as identified by occupational therapists, ie performance/skill deficits. Regardless of diagnosis, performance dysfunction is treated similarly.

Recommended Reading

Allen, C. (1985). *Occupational Therapy for Psychiatric Diseases: Measurement and Management of Cognitive Disabilities*. Boston: Little Brown & Co.

Barris, R., Kielhofner, G., & Watts, J.H. (1989). *Psychosocial Occupational Therapy*. Thorofare, NJ: Slack, Inc.

Bruce, M.A., & Borg, B. (1988). *Frames of Reference in Psychosocial Occupational Therapy*. Thorofare, NJ: Slack, Inc.

References

Allen, C. (1985). *Occupational Therapy for Psychiatric Diseases: Measurement and Management of Cognitive Disabilities*. Boston: Little, Brown & Co.

American Occupational Therapy Association. (1989). *Uniform Terminology Checklist*. Rockville, MD: Author.

Antonosky, A. (1972). Breakdown: A needed fourth step in the conceptual armamentarium of modern medicine. *Social Science and Medicine, 6*, 537-544.

Ayres, A. J. (1972). *Sensory Integration and Learning Disorders*. Los Angeles: Western Psychological Services.

Bruce, M.A. & Borg, B. (1988). *Frames of Reference in Psychosocial Occupational Therapy*. Thorofare, NJ: Slack, Inc.

Kielhofner, G. (1983). *Health Through Occupation: Theory and Practice in Occupational Therapy*. Philadelphia: F.A. Davis

Klerman, G. L. (1988). Classification and DSM-III-R. In A.M. Nicholi (ed.), The New Harvard Guide to Psychiatry. Cambridge MA: Belknap Press, pp. 70-87.

Meyer, A. (1977). The philosophy of occupational therapy. *American Journal of Occupational Therapy, 31*, 639-642.

Porter, R. (1987). *A Social History of Madness*. New York: Weidenfeld & Nicolson.

Reed, K. & Sanderson, S.R. (1980). *Concepts of Occupational Therapy*. Baltimore: Williams & Wilkins.

Rogers, J.C. (1982). Order and disorder in medicine and occupational therapy. *American Journal of Occupational Therapy, 36*, 29-35.

Rogers, J.C. (1983). The study of human occupation. In G. Kielhofner (Ed.), *Health Through Occupation: Theory and Practice in Occupational Therapy*. Philadelphia: F.A. Davis, pp. 93-124.

Spitzer, R.L., Skodal, A.E., Gibbon, M., & Williams, J.B.W. (1988). *Psychopathology: A Casebook*. New York: McGraw-Hill.

Szasz, T. (1974). *The Myth of Mental Illness*, 2nd ed. New York: Harper & Row.

Chapter 3
Disorders of Infancy, Childhood and Adolescence

These disorders are characterized by onset in the early years of life. Although they typically appear early, many are lifelong problems, making the functional implications of this diagnostic group quite significant. The disorders may be present at birth, as in the case of some types of mental retardation, or may appear in adolescence, as is typical of anorexia nervosa. Figure 3-1 lists the diagnoses to be discussed in this chapter.

Figure 3-1
Disorders of Infancy, Childhood & Adolescence

```
Developmental Disorders:
    Mental Retardation
    Pervasive Developmental Disorders: Autistic Disorder
                                        Attention-deficit Hyperactivity Disorder
                                          (ADHD)
                                        Conduct Disorder

Anxiety Disorders of Childhood or Adolescence

Eating Disorders:
    Anorexia Nervosa
    Bulimia Nervosa
```

Diagnoses listed in other categories and covered in later chapters (e.g. depression) may also be applied to children or adolescents. These are disorders that most typically emerge during adulthood, but may occur earlier. Thus, although age of onset is an important factor in differential diagnosis, it is one of many that must be considered.

Childhood and adolescence are characterized by numerous stresses that may lead to disorders not specifically listed in this section. Depression, suicidal ideation or action, substance abuse, adjustment disorders, and sexual acting out are not uncommon. Some theorists suggest that these difficulties may be part of normal development, particularly during adolescence (Freud, 1958). This view is supported by those who feel that modern society presents more difficult dilemmas than existed in earlier times, among these parental divorce, early placement in day care, and peer pressure to use drugs and alcohol (Nicholi, 1988).

This view has been disputed, however. Some researchers have found adolescents to be largely well adjusted (Offer, Marcus, & Offer, 1970). The evidence about children is unclear. It appears, for example, that approximately 10% to 20% of children with divorced families develop long term functional problems (Jellinek & Herzog, 1988), whereas others appear to do as well as their peers. Disputes about what constitutes "normal" childhood and adolescence and what brings about dysfunction await resolution through further research.

The issue of what is normal and what represents dysfunction severe enough to warrant diagnosis must be considered in examining the disorders of infancy, childhood, and adolescence. Although *DSM-III-R* has attempted to be quite specific about the symptoms that must be present for a diagnosis to be made, there remains an element of subjectivity, which some practitioners suggest is particularly problematic where the young are concerned. *DSM-III-R* has been criticized for failing to acknowledge issues about development of personality, sources of information about the child, and so on (Jellinek & Herzog, 1988).

As with all psychiatric diagnoses, those of childhood and adolescence may occur independently or in conjunction with other problems. It is important to note that some of the diagnoses are made on Axis II, for example, mental retardation. These disorders are pervasive throughout the life of the individual. Other disorders, diagnosed on Axis I, are thought to be more time limited although, as will be seen, this is a somewhat artificial distinction. This chapter reviews the diagnostic categories most likely to be seen by occupational therapists. The complete list of diagnoses can be found in Appendix A.

Developmental Disorders

These diagnoses are made on Axis II, as they usually represent lifelong syndromes. They are characterized by deficits in adaptive skills, some of them global, others, like academic skills disorder, specific to a particular type of ability. A careful distinction must be made between small or temporary developmental lags and those that are severe or long-term. Diagnosis must sometimes be deferred until the chronicity of the problem can be documented and its impact on performance confirmed. For example, a child who has a number of medical problems, even as minor as frequent colds, may be delayed briefly but will catch up as soon as the medical problems are resolved. In this case, a diagnosis of developmental delay would not be made.

Mental Retardation

Three characteristics must be present for this diagnosis: subaverage intelligence, deficits in adaptive functioning, and both of which appear prior to age 18. Intelligence (IQ) is usually measured on any of the standard intelligence tests such as the Stanford-Binet or Weschler Intelligence Scale for Children (Zimmerman & Woo-Sam, 1984), with 70 being the score used to define retardation. This cutoff is arbitrary, and IQ tests typically have standard errors of roughly ±4 points. This means that on a given day, a person might score as many as 4 points above or below the score during testing on another day. This is a reflection of the approximate nature of any test score. Thus, the diagnosis must be made cautiously. Children who are retarded achieve developmental milestones later and more slowly than others and may stop developing earlier. For instance, the child might sit at 1 year, walk at 2, say a first word at 3, and ultimately may achieve at maximum the vocabulary of a normal 8 year-old.

Etiology and Incidence

The etiology of retardation is well-established in some cases, but not in others. Some genetic disorders, trisomy 21 (Down's syndrome), for example, cause retardation, as will some prenatal problems such as prenatal malnutrition or fetal alcohol syndrome. A variety of physical problems during early childhood may also lead to retardation, including exposure to toxic substances such as lead (Bellinger, Leviton, Waternaux, Needleman, & Rabinowitz, 1987; Hammond & Beliles, 1980), diseases such as meningitis, and injury, especially head trauma.

Environmental factors may also contribute to retardation. Absence of adequate stimulation or parental deprivation may lead to slowed development and low IQ. Early malnutrition is also a factor (Galler, Ramsey, Solimano, & Lowell, 1983). Bijou (1966) suggests that retardation may occur as a result of inadequate or faulty reinforcement systems for learning, an explanation that reflects behaviorist principles. Biological, environmental, and behavioral factors may interact to exacerbate the deficits of a retarded child. Bijou (1966) further notes that existing explanations of retardation are not entirely satisfactory, and *DSM-III-R* indicates that as many as 40% of cases do not fit any of the known etiological categories.

It appears that mental retardation is present in approximately 1% of the population of the United States and is 50% more common in males (APA, 1987).

Prognosis

Prognosis is, to some extent, dependent on cause. In some instances, retardation may be reversed when the cause of the retardation is removed. Absence of environmental stimulation, for example, may result in failure to thrive (Bullard, Glaser, Heagarty, & Pivchik, 1967). If parents can be taught to make the environment more stimulating, the retardation may be remediated and the child returned to normal function. Some government programs, such as Project Head Start, appear to have positive effects on IQ for many children who are somewhat delayed developmentally (these programs were not designed for mentally retarded children, however).

Similarly, where a biological cause can be established, medical treatment of the underlying problem may prevent retardation from worsening, although generally speaking the existing damage will be permanent. For example, if retardation is the result of lead toxicity, agents may be introduced to remove lead from the system. This treatment will prevent further damage, but will generally not reverse damage that has already occurred (Galler et al., 1983). Prompt treatment of diseases such as meningitis, when such treatment exists, may also minimize the probability of retardation or limit damage.

In most cases, however, IQ is quite stable throughout the life span (Zimmerman & Woo-Sam, 1984). Thus, intellectual capacity is unlikely to change in most retarded individuals. Functional ability may be remediated, however, the most interventions with retarded individuals focus on some form of education or training. This may include behavior modification (Bijou, 1966) or any of a variety of educational approaches. Depending on degree of retardation, the individual may be taught to cook simple meals, to dress and maintain personal hygiene, and perform simple vocational tasks, making some individuals relatively independent and self-sufficient.

It should be mentioned that education may extend to the family, both for purposes of prevention (educating pregnant women about the need for good nutrition, for example) and for management of the retarded child. It should also be noted that although function may be remediated, individuals who are retarded by definition do not achieve the same level as their nonretarded peers.

Depending on the degree of impairment, institutionalization may become necessary. Individuals who are profoundly retarded may be unable to learn the skills necessary to enable them to live even in sheltered environments. For many less severely impaired individuals, however, many types of sheltered environments, special schools, and, later, supervised independent living situations, such as group homes, may provide alternatives to institutionalization.

Implications for Function and Treatment

Retardation may be classified as mild (IQ 55 to 70), moderate (IQ 40 to 55), severe (IQ 25 to 40), or profound (IQ below 25). These are approximate ranges, but they provide a rough guide to expected function. Although IQ and functional ability are correlated, it is recognized that a variety of factors may affect the functional picture presented by individuals with similar IQ scores. There has been much discussion, for example, about the possibility of cultural bias of IQ tests (Zimmerman & Woo-Sam, 1984), which might cause a low score in someone who otherwise has a reasonable level of function. In fact, there has been much controversy around this point, with some researchers feeling that IQ tests should not be used to identify retardation. As an example, some children from deprived backgrounds may know a great deal of street jargon, but have limited vocabularies for English words used in the larger society that appear on some IQ tests.

Generally, individuals who have low IQs show performance deficits in most areas of function. These may present as delays in the development of specific abilities, the absence of some abilities, or deficits in the skill with which activities are performed. For example, a retarded child might sit relatively late, might not sit at all, or might sit with poor control and posture. A profoundly retarded individual may never acquire speech or learn to feed him or herself, whereas a mildly retarded individual may learn to read and do simple arithmetic problems.

Except where there are obvious physical signs of retardation at birth, such as in the case of trisomy 21, it is the functional delays observed by parents that are most likely to result in the identification of retarded individuals. Parents typically become concerned when a child does not sit, walk, or talk at the expected time.

Functional deficits tend to be pervasive, though as with all children, some areas may be more delayed than others. A retarded child is likely to have motor, social, cognitive, sensory, and psychological deficits, though he or she may have relatively less motor delay than cognitive delay, or less social delay than motor delay. For example, some children who are retarded may be quite sociable, but have difficulty with academic skills. Deficits are also roughly correlated with IQ, so that a profoundly retarded child is likely to have severely impaired function in all areas. Deficits will be noted in all areas of function: play, social interaction, activities of daily living (ADL), and education. These translate into later deficits in work, play, leisure, and ADL/IADL (instrumental activities of daily living). ADL includes basic self-care: feeding, bathing, toileting, dressing. IADL includes higher level self-care such as cooking, shopping, managing money, cleaning a house, and so on.

Intervention is generally medical and educational/behavioral. Medical treatment focuses on reversing treatable conditions and maximizing health to preserve intact function. Ear infections, sore throats, etc., may add to functional impairment and must be treated. Provision of adequate nutrition and exercise and monitoring of health in individuals unable to report symptoms is vital to optimal functioning.

For children, educational approaches are most often employed. For those with mild impairment, "mainstreaming," inclusion to the greatest degree possible in the regular school system, is the intervention of choice. These children may have special classes during the course of the day and attend regular classes when possible. Those more severely impaired will attend special schools.

Behavioral interventions can be valuable both for children and adults. Enhanced social and vocational function can be obtained by carefully outlining the steps involved in each task, and then providing reinforcement as the individual accomplishes each step. A child might need information and practice to manage a simple social interaction that includes "hello," "how are you?" Less attention has been paid to leisure performance, but there is every reason to believe that this, too, can be enhanced through behavioral and educational approaches. The environment in which treatment occurs is important (Shah & Holmes, 1987), with sheltered living in the community being successful in promoting optimal performance in moderately retarded individuals. Schalock, Harper, and Carver (1981) suggest that the benefit can be maximized when individuals receive focused training prior to placement. Among mildly to moderately retarded individuals with mild functional impairment, they found that 55 of 69 placements of adult mentally retarded individuals were successful following structured training. Most of their subjects had jobs and friends.

Such specifically targeted skill training programs, among them social and vocational interventions, appear to have positive outcomes. Matson (1981) reported that independence training is quite effective. Interventions targeted to motor, sensory, and sensory motor skills have also been undertaken, though with less clear cut success. These include play activities, listening to music, and paper and pencil activities, among others.

It is important to note, however, that although many types of treatment appear to promote optimal function, none completely reverses retardation, except cases where it is medically possible to do so. On the other hand, recent evidence suggests that some types of retardation (trisomy 21, for instance) have better prognoses than assumed in the past. Some of these individuals achieve quite good function, and many report very positive levels of life satisfaction. They may, for example, become socially adept, learn to read and do arithmetic at a fairly basic level, and hold jobs. One such individual became a teachers' aide in a program for retarded children.

Implications for Occupational Therapy

For individuals who are retarded, the goal of treatment is most often habilitation (enabling) rather than rehabilitation, since they must acquire skills they never had rather than regain those lost. Impairment tends to be consistent across skills and, therefore, across performance.

In general, goals of occupational therapy focus on enabling maximal performance. This requires careful assessment of both deficits and strengths. Individuals who are retarded often wish to do the same activities as their peers (Edgerton, 1976) and are able to accomplish many developmental milestones, albeit more slowly than their peers. Although recognition of strengths is important in working with any client group, it is particularly vital with these individuals as it is easy to despair.

At the same time, realistic appraisal is necessary. The realities of the starting point for a particular individual cannot be overlooked, and the duration of the learning process for a particular skill may place limits on eventual achievement.

Profoundly retarded individuals are unlikely to acquire more than extremely minimal skills. Early intervention may need to focus on eating and on movement to facilitate dressing in much the same way a therapist might approach a child with severe cerebral palsy (Carrasco & Powell, 1989). Sensory integration and sensory stimulation may be of value.

With children who are less severely retarded, training and education may prove quite valuable, particularly when practice is built in. For example, body awareness may facilitate dressing skills. In one school, children aged 6 to 10 years spent several weeks playing "Simon Says," pointing to body parts on dolls, doing the "Hokey Pokey" ("you put your left foot in..."), and so on. Two months later, they were ready to begin putting legs into pant legs, arms into sleeves. It should be noted that sensory stimulation is also a component of these activities.

Identifying leisure activities at which they can succeed is also important for these children. Many have siblings they would like to emulate, but Little League may be beyond them unless leagues are specially organized.

As these children age, vocational training and training in independent living skills become increasingly important (Anthony, 1979). This includes training in social skills and sex education. Although individuals who are retarded may desire the same activities as their nonretarded peers, they tend to conceptualize at a concrete level. Since many will live independently or in semi-sheltered environments they need to understand the accompanying responsibilities. One young woman, for example, expressed a wish for a child until she sat through an independent living group while a baby-doll cried in the background. Another young man planned to go to the movies every day until the therapist had him put his pay from the sheltered workshop in piles to represent rent, food, transportation, etc.

In general, for both children and adults, sensory stimulation may be of value, as will presenting tasks in small steps that can be practiced in sequence (Martin, 1989). An additional focus must be on self-esteem, since these individuals often compare themselves negatively to others, and often confront perjorative comments by others. Mainstreamed children, for example, must contend with schoolmates who call them "moron" or "dummy."

As can be inferred from this discussion, treatment may occur in a variety of sites, including the home, a special school, a regular school, an institution, a sheltered workshop, or a supervised living facility (Martin, 1989). Each requires sensitivity on the part of the therapist to the needs of the client in that setting and the possibility of movement from setting to setting. Children nearing the end of the educational process may need intensive work on vocational and job related skills.

Pervasive Developmental Disorders

Autism

This is a rare condition that represents the most severe manifestation of Pervasive Developmental Disorder. Because of the extreme nature of the deficits with which it is associated, it has received considerable notice. A number of popular books (Greenfield, 1986) have brought it to the attention of the general population. For the diagnosis to be made, social interaction, communication, and activity must be impaired. These children have severe social deficits, lack speech, or have peculiar speech patterns, and have unusual stereotyped movements like hand flapping. Typical autistic children may sit without making eye contact or speaking while engaging in some self-stimulating behavior, possibly spinning their bodies or twirling their hair for hours on end. Autism often occurs in the presence of other disorders, particularly mental retardation.

Etiology and Incidence

The etiology of autism is increasingly well understood. At one point it was considered a problem of inadequate parenting, believed to be associated with maternal coldness or rejection. This idea has been discredited, and current hypotheses center on the possibility of some sort of neurological dysfunction. It is known, for example, that autistic children have poor receptive language and symbol use (Atlas, 1987), supporting the notion of central nervous system (CNS) deficits. There is a growing body of evidence that autism is a neurological disorder.

Incidence is estimated at 4 to 5 per 10,000 population (Jellinek & Herzog, 1988). The disorder is three times as frequent in males.

Prognosis

Prognosis is considered poor (Jellinek & Herzog, 1988) largely because of the pervasive nature of the disorder and its unclear etiology. Although some individuals may show unpredictable improvements, the majority continue to be fairly impaired throughout life. In particular, social impairment and behavioral and psychiatric symptoms have been found to persist (Rumsey, Rapoport, & Scheery, 1985). Factors that help predict long term outcomes include IQ and speech abilities at age 5.

Some studies have shown gradual improvement in symptoms. However, Rumsey and colleagues (1985) studied 14 autistic individuals, 9 of whom were considered high functioning, and found that all had ongoing social and occupational impairment. Skill and performance are globally and chronically affected although improvement may occur.

Implications for Function and Treatment

Autistic individuals show extreme impairments in social functioning, ability to communicate, and in performance of most activities. These impairments are often characterized by peculiarities in performance, as well as absence of performance. For example, an autistic individual may be able to speak, but may put words together in ways that are not meaningful to others. He or she may repeat jingles from television commercials all day, or simply repeat meaningless phrases. Similarly, he or she may be able to perform specific fine motor tasks, but be unable to put them together into a meaningful sequence of activities to accomplish a specific goal. He or she might move pegs back and forth on a table without ever putting them in a peg-board or making a picture.

The deficits in function usually preclude most forms of normal goal oriented occupation. Autistic individuals are often unable to perform ADL and IADL activities, have disturbed patterns of play, and are unable to study and, later, to work. More functional individuals with this disability may be able to do simple tasks such as dressing, but do them in a rigid and ritualistic fashion (e.g., always wearing a certain type of clothing, buttoning a specific button first, etc.). Communication skills are particularly poor (Atlas, 1987) and may, in fact, provide diagnostic clues to the disorder. The child may mutter a single phrase all day, or parrot back whatever is said. Because the etiology is as yet unclear, treatment is not well-established. Most interventions currently employed are behavioral, with a focus on speech development, increasing behaviors such as ADL skills, or decreasing undesirable behaviors such as peculiar movements. More and more autistic children are in public schools, often in special classes, although the majority of programs are still provided at special schools or in inpatient settings, as they are usually designed to provide high levels of input throughout the day.

Behavior modification has been employed for specific deficits. One study focused on affectionate behavior (McEvoy, Nordquist, Twardosz, Heckaman, Wehby, & Denny, 1988), reporting on an effort to teach autistic children to express positive emotion to those around them. The authors reported that some very limited improvement was found. Because of the severity of dysfunction, behavioral programs usually focus on small components of performance, making global improvement an extremely long term goal. Environmental enrichment with sensory stimulation has been employed with some success in an effort to provide more general intervention (Ward, 1985).

Implications for Occupational Therapy

Because autistic children are so severely impaired, observation must often substitute for formal assessment, and treatment goals must be sensitive to the probability that change will occur in very small steps.

Ideally, adaptive behavior, cognitive, motor, and perceptual skills should be evaluated (Nelson, 1980), but this often proves difficult because of the profound communication deficits so characteristic of these children.

Many of the intervention strategies used with severely and profoundly retarded children, including sensory stimulation and sensory integration, may be attempted (Herman, 1980).   In general, focus will be on basic self-care and communication. Motivation and attention are key issues. Behavioral techniques may be helpful both in enhancing attention and in training autistic children to perform sequences of activities related to self-care.

Disruptive Behavior Disorders

These diagnoses are made on Axis I. They represent disorders of behavior that may initially be more disturbing to others than to the individual. However, the presence of these disorders may have long-term effects on self-esteem and social participation, as the individual is likely to receive considerable social censure and rejection as a result of his or her behavior.   In addition, behaviors may interfere with learning, causing long term academic problems.

Attention-Deficit Hyperactivity Disorder (ADHD)

This disorder is characterized by excessive inattention, impulsiveness, and hyperactivity. Typically, the child has difficulty attending to others and is extremely active physically. Problematic behaviors, including at least eight specific symptoms of inattention, impulsiveness, or hyperactivity, must be present for at least 6 months for the diagnosis to be made. The behaviors must be judged to be more severe than in normal children, a criterion that presents significant diagnostic difficulties, as noted below. The problem behaviors must appear prior to age 7 to be diagnosed as ADHD.

The diagnosis is problematic, as individual adult tolerance for activity in children varies. What is labeled "youthful exuberence" in some families may be intolerable to other parents. In some children, the diagnosis is not made until the school years, when ADHD may interfere with ability to complete school work. In other instances, the diagnosis may be made on the basis of the adult's difficulty accepting the behavior, rather than on clearly disturbed behavior on the part of the child. Many times, however, these children are easily recognizable. They respond to the slightest distraction, running to chase dust, sunlight, and every small sound, rather than focusing on the task at hand. Their level of activity is often exhausting just to watch and their distractability makes them hard to discipline or manage. One child frequently rode his bike at high speed into the street, across neighbors' gardens without regard for safety.

Etiology and Incidence

Etiology of ADHD is not clearly established, although it is suspected that it may occur in the presence of neurological damage or a disordered central nervous system. First described by Hoffman in 1926, it was originally called Minimal Brain Damage (MBD). Later it was known as hyperkenesis, then hyperactivity (Rutter, & Taylor, 1978). Current theories suggest that the problem is one of CNS organization (Jellinek & Herzog, 1988). Children with ADHD have been found to be more field dependent than others (Stoner & Glynn, 1987). This means that they have difficulty separating figures from the background in pictures, a difficulty that would contribute, among other things, to reading difficulties and problems with visual discrimination tasks and inability to filter out normal distractions. They also have more frequent language disorders than other children (Love & Thompson, 1988), supporting the idea of CNS disturbance. The disorder also seems to be more common in families where other relatives have had the diagnosis, suggesting a familial or genetic component.

This is a common disorder, possibly occurring in 3% of the population (APA, 1987). It is much more common in males.

Prognosis

Prognosis is good for some of these children. Many children seem to "outgrow" the disorder as they get older. Satterfield and Satterfield (1981) found this to be the case in their investigation of 100 subjects. They noted that treatment improves the probability of a positive outcome. In addition, medications are effective in some instances in minimizing the effects of the disorder. A potential negative consequence of ADHD is the possibility that the child will become depressed or develop low self-esteem as a result of the social disapproval or academic difficulties that often accompany the disorder. Understandably, the prognosis is less favorable if ADHD is accompanied by retardation or some other behavioral disorder (e.g., conduct disorder) (August, Stewart, & Holmes, 1983). Hechtman, Weiss, & Perlman (1980) found ongoing problems with heterosexual relationships, assertiveness, and self-esteem. Other studies note persistent school difficulties and the possibility of emerging antisocial behavior (August et al, 1980).

Implications for Function and Treatment

Children with ADHD are able to function in many areas. They are usually able to perform ADL and some IADL activities, to play and to interact with peers on some level. Generally speaking, social and academic performance are most impaired. Peers and adults may find the excessive activity and difficulty concentrating annoying, and avoid or chastize the child. These children are often unpopular with peers because of their poor self control - grabbing toys, disrupting games, etc. In some instances, poor impulse control leads the child to behave in socially inappropriate or antisocial fashion, again leading to disapproval or legal difficulties.

In the academic sphere, poor concentration and impulse control present significant problems. Not only is learning impaired, but teachers find these children difficult, compounding their learning problems. They often do poorly in school and then become anxious about their performance, exacerbating their learning difficulties. Other activities that require concentration or attention may be difficult or impossible for these children, limiting the play and leisure activities in which they are able to participate.

Medication is sometimes used to control ADHD. Amphetamines, Ritalin in particular, are often used. The exact mechanism by which they work is not established, but they seem effective in reducing hyperactive behavior. They may have the effect of increasing attention level. There is some controversy about the use of these drugs, as their long-term effects are not thought to be adequately understood. In addition, some researchers believe that they are used too freely, particularly in cases where the diagnosis may be marginal. Most important, a review of more than 100 studies suggests that effectiveness of the drugs is not clear (Barkley, 1977). It seems that positive effects result in more manageable behavior rather than improved academic performance (Barkley & Cunningham, 1978). For this reason, there has been concern that the drugs are "abused" in the sense that they provide relief for the adult, while some less intrusive approach might be equally effective for the child.

Other interventions are both behavioral and environmental. Behavioral approaches attempt to reinforce efforts to concentrate and control hyperactivity. Environmental approaches are used to design low stimulus environments in which distractions are kept to a minimum.

Robinson, Newby, and Ganzell (1981) report positive outcomes using a token system. Kendall and Finch (1978) report that cognitive-behavioral interventions are effective. These mix education information with behavioral intervention. In addition, there is evidence that parent training may reduce problem behavior in the child by providing the parent with a range of interventions to help manage the child's hyperactive behavior (Atkeson & Forehand, 1978).

Implications for Occupational Therapy

As the name of the disorder implies, attention is an important factor in working with these children. Several approaches may be useful. Clearly, environmental structuring to minimize distraction may help. Occupational therapy may also provide patterned, sequenced sensory input to attempt to help the child better organize his or her surroundings. Both relaxation (Kwako, 1980) and perceptual motor training (Christ, 1980) have been reported as helpful.

In addition, self-esteem is an important issue for these children. Identification of activities they can do well can be enormously helpful in convincing them, often despite repeated scoldings from exasperated adults, that they do have strengths.

Conduct Disorder

This diagnosis is made if, within 6 months of being seen for evaluation, the individual has engaged in at least three episodes of serious problem behavior, such as truancy, stealing, lying, or cruelty to animals. The diagnosis may be made in adults who do not meet the criteria for antisocial personality, but is more typically made in individuals under age 18. There are two subtypes: aggressive, characterized by social isolation, and group delinquent type, characterized by occurrence of antisocial behavior that is part of group membership (Jellinek & Herzog, 1988).

Etiology and Incidence

Etiology of this disorder is not clearly established, although there is speculation that, like antisocial personality, it may be the result of either inconsistent or overprotective parenting. Behaviorists suggest that the result of these parental reactions is poor understanding of the consequences of behavior, whereas psychodynamic theorists suggest that there is poor development or integration of the superego. In addition, environmental and socioeconomic explanations have been advanced, suggesting that this behavior is the result of deprivation or an environment that supports or encourages acting out. It occurs frequently in combination with disorders like ADHD, and it has been suggested that it may be a consequence of the CNS damage or the negative appraisals of self that occur as a result of the accompanying condition.

This disorder occurs in roughly 9% of males and 2% of females (APA, 1987). Between 10% and 15% of children referred for psychiatric treatment have this diagnosis (Jellinek & Herzog, 1988).

Prognosis

Milder forms of the disorder seem to have reasonably good prognoses, whereas the more severe form predicts later delinquent and adult antisocial behavior (Faretra, 1981; Robins, 1978). As the disorder coexists with others, including enuresis (Faretra, 1981), retardation, ADHD, depression, and substance abuse, if the coexisting condition is remediated, the conduct disorder may also improve. Similarly, if the environment is altered or improved, symptoms may subside. However, when there are coexisting conditions the prognosis is worse (August et al, 1980).

Patterson (1979) provides a comprehensive review of outcome studies and concludes that these disorders tend to be stable over time, and that children who steal are likely to commit other offenses. He notes, however, that those with other behavioral manifestations of conduct disorder are not especially likely to turn to stealing. In general, fewer and milder symptoms and later onset are predictive of better outcomes as are good school performance, availability of good parenting, and having no delinquent friends (Robins, 1970). For those individuals for whom the conduct disorder is evident primarily in group situations, removing the child from the disordered group reduces the problematic behavior. This is a more tractable form of the disorder.

Implications for Function and Treatment

Many of these individuals have difficulty with school or work performance, possibly as the result of cognitive or attention deficits, possibly as a result of attitudinal problems (Patterson, 1979). As a rule, ADL and IADL functions are not impaired. Leisure and play tend to focus on socially unacceptable activities, as acting out may take the place of more normal endeavors. The child may spend after school time shoplifting, or may cut school and spend the time setting fires in trash cans.

These children are more likely to have social difficulties and to be delinquent (Roff & Wirt, 1984). They solve their frequent interpersonal disputes with fights or by banding together with other socially maladept children. Recent reports of "wilding" are an example of the group form of conduct disorder. Some of the social problems may stem from poor ability to detect and understand social cues from others (Dodge, 1983; Dodge, Murphy, & Bushsbaum, 1984), leading to speculation that training in these skills might improve function and reduce symptoms.

Glasser (1975) recommended a type of milieu therapy, which he labeled reality therapy, as a mechanism for making individuals accountable for their behavior. This is one of many milieu treatments that have been attempted, including the behavioral approach of the token economy, with rewards or reinforcements for acceptable behavior. Milieu treatments are those in which the entire environment is carefully structured to have therapeutic impact. Behavior modification has been reported successful to some extent (Patterson, 1979), producing something in the range of a 30% decrease in undesireable behaviors. There is also evidence that as family discord decreases, delinquency decreases (Rutter & Hersov, 1985), suggesting that family therapy or marital therapy for the parents of such a child may be useful.

Implications for Occupational Therapy

Occupational therapists may work with children with conduct disorders in several ways. First, energy may be channeled to more appropriate activities, with copious reinforcement for acceptable behavior. Expectations for behavior during such activities must be carefully identified and reasonable positive or negative outcomes systematically provided.

Second, self-esteem of these children must be considered. Experiences of success can be of great value in building a more positive self-concept.

Finally, opportunities for expression must be provided. Many of these children come from disturbed environments. They may be unable to express feelings adequately and may do better through play.

At the same time, the possibility of coexisting deficits must be considered. ADHD should be addressed, as should other disorders.

Anxiety Disorders

There are several anxiety disorders in children, all typified by anxiety or panic particularly related to threatened separation from familiar caretakers or presence of unfamiliar adults. Duration prior to diagnosis may be from 2 weeks (separation anxiety disorder) to 6 months or more (overanxious disorder).

Etiology and Incidence

It is suspected that anxiety disorders occur more commonly in children with developmental disorders, such as academic skills disorder. It is also possible that anxiety is the result of premature separation from the primary caretaker (Bowlby, 1969).

All the anxiety disorders are fairly common and occur with equal frequency in males and females (APA, 1987). The exception is Avoidant Disorder of Childhood, which, although common, is somewhat more frequent in females.

Prognosis

In some instances, the disorder disappears spontaneously, sometimes after only one episode. In other cases, it may become severe and disabling, as the individual may develop a social phobia or school phobia, and refuse to leave the home. The child may have a stomachache every morning, or cry and scream when the school bus comes. Remediation is easiest in those situations where there are clear environmental factors, such as excessive pressure to perform well in school, contributing to the problem. Altering the environment may be quite effective in those situations. One child got sick at school every morning before computer class. She improved when she received individual tutoring that convinced her she could handle the work.

Implications for Function and Treatment

As noted, in severe cases school, social, and leisure activities may be severely compromised. Individuals may become so anxious at the thought of having to perform in one of these spheres that they become physically ill. ADL activities are usually not affected, nor are IADL activities that may be performed in the home. However, activities that require interaction with strangers or leaving familiar environments may be all but impossible. It appears to be performance (i.e., school and leisure activity) rather than motor, social, or other skills that is impaired.

Treatment is not well understood, although some theorists suspect that altering home circumstances to provide a more stable, less pressuring environment may be helpful. A parent who is a sports enthusiast may need to learn to let his or her little leaguer just enjoy the game. Some behavioral techniques are also attempted, although such methods as systematic desensitization, which are helpful with some anxious adults, may be too complex for young children.

Implications for Occupational Therapy

Relaxation techniques may be helpful to children with anxiety disorders. Using mental imagery to imagine success, enjoyment, and relaxation can provide a useful prelude to anxiety provoking activities.

In addition, activities can in themselves be relaxing, particularly if those that are enjoyable to the child can be identified. Sometimes pairing a pleasant activity with one that evokes anxiety can relieve feelings of distress. The student who felt sick before computer class did well when the task was playing computer games rather than doing schoolwork on the computer. The positive association later generalized to other computer activities.

Expressive arts may be beneficial as a way to uncover and explore fears. A child who was afraid to leave his room drew pictures of enormous snakes and spiders. It turned out he had encountered a snake in his basement that had greatly frightened him. It was then possible to address his fear.

Eating Disorders

The two major disorders in this group, anorexia nervosa and bulimia nervosa, have received a great deal of attention in recent years, perhaps because they seem to be increasingly common. Anorexia is characterized by a refusal to gain weight, fear of gaining weight, and belief that they are overweight in individuals who are, in fact, significantly below acceptable body weight for their height. It is not unusual to hear women with anorexia who look emaciated claim to be obese. In women, amenorrhea is also present. Bulimia is characterized by a binge/purge cycle in individuals who are more likely to be of normal weight or overweight. The purging is accomplished through induced vomiting or the use of laxatives, and the entire cycle is accompanied by a sense of loss of control of eating. Binging and purging occurs frequently, at least twice a week, and must persist over at least 3 months before the diagnosis is made. Bulimics are excessively concerned about weight.

Etiology and Incidence

To some extent, these disorders are cultural, as thinness is considered desirable. Vocation may also correlate with anorexia, as ballet dancers, for example, are very likely to suffer from bulimia or anorexia (Herzog, 1988). Bruch (1973) hypothesized that obesity and anorexia stemmed from issues of maternal control. The family has been implicated as the source of the disorder by others as well (Minuchin, Roseman, & Baker, 1978). Some suggest that anorexia is likely to occur in families where expectations are high for performance. A variety of biological changes occur in individuals with anorexia and bulimia, leading some to suggest that the cause is biological (Herzog, 1988; Kaye, Ebert, Gwirtsman, & Weiss, 1984). It is difficult, however, to know whether eating changes cause the biological changes or vice versa. Menstruation is affected in anorexics, and abnormal brain serotonergic metabolism has been found in both anorexics and bulimics (Kaye et al, 1984).

Anorexics' disturbed body image, absence of concern about the problem, overactivity, and inability to recognize hunger led Bruch (1962) to speculate that these individuals have a perceptual disorder.

Examination of bulimics has identified similarities between this disorder and substance abuse on Minnesota Multiphasic Personality Inventory profiles (Hatsukami, Owen, Pyle & Mitchell, 1982) suggesting that this is another form of substance abuse disorder. Binging may cause a short term "high" encouraging the behavior (Kaye, Gwirtsman, George, Weiss & Jimerson, 1986). For some women it may begin as a rather social behavior. A roommate might share the "secret of success" for dieting, for example, or sorority sisters might down dozens of doughnuts every Saturday morning, then take laxatives.

It now appears that approximately 10% to 15% of American women have one of these syndromes (Pope, Hudson & Yurgelun-Todd, 1984). Approximately 90% to 95% of cases occur in women.

Prognosis

It has been estimated that between 5% and 23% of anorexics ultimately die of the disorder (Pope et al., 1984). In some cases, only one episode of several weeks or months duration occurs, after which weight and eating return to normal. In others, however, the disorder is chronic.

Hsu, Crisp and Harding (1979) reported that approximately 50% of anorexics had good long-term outcomes. Outcome appeared related to age at onset and severity of symptoms, with earlier onset having worse prognosis and milder symptoms, better prognosis. Morgan and Russell (1975) found that their subjects could be divided roughly by thirds into those with good, fair and poor outcomes. Norman and Herzog (1984) found persistent functional difficulties particularly related to social interaction and activity related to food in a one year follow-up of 40 patients.

Implications for Function and Treatment

Anorexics often have good vocational function (Cantwell, Sturzenberg, Burroughs, Salkin & Green, 1976). A follow-up study of 100 women found 80 employed four to eight years after diagnosis (Hsu et al., 1979). Social functioning, however, tends to be poor, as these individuals are often isolated and asexual. Estimates range from as low as 22% to as high as 73% having satisfactory social functioning on a long-term basis. One study reported 60% to have good sexual adjustment, and 50% good socioeconomic adjustment (Morgan & Russell, 1975). The figures are quite variable, leading to some confusion about the exact nature of long-term function in anorexics (Herzog, Keller & Lavori, 1988).

ADL and IADL are generally not affected, except in the area of eating and cooking. The term anorexia is somewhat misleading, as these individuals are often obsessed with food and plan their lives around it. One woman spent an hour each morning carefully and ritualistically preparing the lettuce leaf with mustard that constituted her breakfast.

Bulimia appears to be a much more chronic and episodic disorder, often continuing for a lifetime (Herzog, 1982). Although it is not as likely to cause death, a number of serious health problems may result, including digestive disorders and heart and kidney problems. Bulimics are more likely to recognize the need for help and to accept it, but the disease is relatively intractable (Herzog, 1982). Predictors of outcome are not clear (Herzog et al, 1988).

An obsession with food is the key factor interfering with function in bulimics (Herzog, 1982). They are so preoccupied with food and eating that their work may suffer and social activities are often badly affected. These problems are the result of the time taken with obsessing about food, as well as the fear that they will be rejected by anyone who learns of the obsession. As with anorexics, ADL and IADL are not affected, except as they relate to food and its preparation. A woman might spend her work day plotting her evening visits to the ice cream store, pizza parlor, and how she will mask her binge by shopping in a new neighborhood. A variety of treatments has been employed for both anorexics and bulimics. In some cases, anorexics require hospitalization, often as the result of life-threatening weight loss, whereas bulimics are almost always treated in outpatient settings. Behavioral techniques are used both in inpatient and outpatient settings (Garner & Bennis, 1982). In addition, group therapy has been advocated (Brotman, Alonso, & Herzog, 1985), as has family therapy (Schwartz, Barret, & Saba, 1985). The use of antidepressant medications shows promise, particularly in treating anorexics (Pope, Hudson, Jonas, Yurgelun-Todd, 1985). Other recommended approaches include individual psychotherapy, cognitive therapies, education, and self-help groups (Herzog, 1988).

Implications for Occupational Therapy

As with so many psychiatric disorders, self-esteem is a particular problem for anorexic and bulimic individuals. Anorexics report feeling ineffective (McCall, Friedland, & Kerr, 1986) and are often perfectionistic. One anorexic college student repeatedly wrote 100-page reports, unable to force herself to do less than perfect work. Success experiences can help modify these feelings.

These perfectionistic traits often are displayed in occupational therapy. An anorexic patient repeatedly attempted a mosaic tile project, noting tiny imperfections in each. Limit setting by the therapist, as well as discussion of the trait, were helpful to that client. Reinforcement of behavioral change helped in this process.

Introduction of new activities to develop new interests may divert attention from food. For both bulimics and anorexics, food is a major focus. These individuals may have few other interests and no friends because of poor social skills. Development of new interests is vital.

Figure 3-2 provides a summary of the diagnostic categories discussed in this chapter. Major symptoms and functional deficits are listed.

Figure 3-2
Developmental Disorders

Disorder	Symptoms	Functional Deficits
Mental Retardation	1. Subaverage intelligence	Global ADL/IADL, work, leisure
	2. Deficits in adaptive function	Global motor, sensory motor, social, cognitive
	3. Appears before age 18	Range from mild to severe
Autistic Disorder	1. Impaired social interaction	Global ADL/IADL, work, leisure
	2. Impaired communication	Global motor, sensory motor, social, cognitive, psychological
	3. Restricted activity repertoire	Usually severe
	4. Onset during infancy or childhood	
Attention Deficit Hyperactive Disorder (ADHD)	1. Restlessness, distractability	Social, school, leisure
	2. Excessive activity	Mild to severe
	3. Impulsivity	Usually improve during adolescence
	4. Onset before age 7	
Conduct Disorder	1. Has engaged in at least 3 antisocial acts within past six months	Social, leisure, school
Anxiety Disorders	1. Extreme anxiety	Social
	2. May be related to separation, or classified as avoidant	Social/leisure

Figure 3-2 *continued*

Disorder	Symptoms	Functional Deficits
Anorexia Nervosa	1. Weight loss to at least 15% below expected body weight, or failure to gain, if still growing	Social, leisure
	2. Intense fear of gaining weight	ADL
	3. Disturbed body image: belief one is too fat although clearly underweight.	May affect work/school
	4. In females, amenorrhea	Possibly sensory, sensory integrative
Bulimia Nervosa	1. Recurrent binge eating	Social, leisure
	2. Sense of lack of control over binges	Possibly work/school
	3. Purging through vomiting, laxatives, etc.	
	4. Occurs at least 2 x/wk for at least 3 months	
	5. Overconcern with body shape	

References

Anthony, W.A. (1979). *The Principles of Psychiatric Rehabilitation*. Amherst, MA: Human Resource Development Press.

Atkeson, B.M. & Forehand, R. (1978). Parent behavioral training for problem children: An examination of studies using multiple outcome measures. *Journal of Abnormal Child Psychology, 6,* 449-460.

Atlas, J.A. (1987). Symbol use by developmentally disabled children. *Psychological Reports, 61,* 207-214.

August, G.J., Stewart, M.A., & Holmes, C.S. (1983). A four-year follow-up of hyperactive boys with and without conduct disorder. *British Journal of Psychiatry, 143,* 192-198.

Barkley, R.A. (1977). A review of stimulant drug research with hyperactive children. *Journal of Child Psychology and Psychiatry, 18*, 137-165.

Barkley, R.A. & Cunningham, C.E. (1978). Do stimulant drugs improve the academic performance of hyperkinetic children?: A review of outcome studies. *Clinical Pediatrics, 17*, 85-92.

Bellinger, D., Leviton, A., Waternaux, C., Needleman, H., & Rabinowitz, M. (1987). Longitudinal analyses of prenatal and postnatal lead exposure and early cognitive development. *New England Journal of Medicine, 316*, 1037-1043.

Bijou, S.W. (1966). A functional analysis of retarded development. In N.R. Ellis (Ed.), *International Review of Research in Mental Retardation*, Vol. 1. New York: Academic Press.

Bowlby, J. (1969). *Attachment and Loss*. New York: Basic Books.

Brotman, A.W., Alonso, A., & Herzog, D.B. (1985). Group therapy for bulimics: Clinical experience and practice recommendations. *Group, 9*, 15-23.

Bruch, H. (1962). Perceptual and conceptual disturbances in anorexia nervosa. *Psychosomatic Medicine, 24*, 187-194

Bruch, H. (1973). *Eating Disorders: Obesity, Anorexia Nervosa, and the Person Within*. New York: Basic Books.

Bullard, D.M., Glaser, H.H., Heagarty, M.C., & Pivcheck, E.C. (1967). Failure to thrive in the neglected child. *American Journal of Orthopsychiatry, 37*, 680-690.

Cantwell, D.P., Sturzenberg, S., Burroughs, J., Salkin, B., & Green, J.K. (1976). Anorexia nervosa: An affective disorder. *Archives of General Psychiatry, 33*, 1039-1044.

Carrasco, R.C., & Powell, N. (1989). Children with cerebral palsy. In Allen, A.S., & Pratt, P.N. (Eds.), *Occupational Therapy for Children* 2nd ed. pp. 396-421.

Christ, P.A.H. (1980). Electromyographic biofeedback and perceptual motor training for hyperactivity. *Occupational Therapy in Mental Health, 1*(:3), 47-57.

Dodge, K.A., Murphy, R.R., & Buchsbaum K. (1984). The assessment of intention-cue detection skills in children: Implications for developmental psychopathology. *Child Development, 55*, 163-173.

Dodge, K.A. (1983). Behavioral antecedents of peer social status. *Child Development, 54*, 1386-1399.

Edgerton, R., & Bercovici, S. (1976). The cloak of competence years later. *American Journal of Mental Deficiency, 80*, 485-497.

Faretra, G. (1981). A profile of aggression from adolescence to adulthood: An 18-year follow-up of psychiatrically disturbed and violent adolescents. *American Journal of Orthopsychiaty, 51*, 439-453.

Freud, A. (1958). Adolescence. *Psychoanalytic Study of Children, 13,* 255-278.

Galler, J.R., Ramsey, F., Solimano, G., & Lowell, W.E. (1983). The influence of early malnutrition on subsequent behavioral development: II. Classroom behavior. *Journal of the American Academy of Child Psychiatry, 22,* 16-22.

Garner, D.M. & Bennis, K.M. (1982) A cognitive-behavioral approach to anorexia nervosa. *Cognitive Therapy Research, 6,* 123-150.

Glasser, W. (1975). *Reality Therapy: A New Approach to Psychiatry.* New York: Perenial Library/Harper & Row.

Greenfield, J. (1986). *A Client Called Noah.* New York: Henry Holt and Co.

Hammond, P.B., & Beliles, R.P. (1980). Metals. In J. Doull, C.D. Klaassen, & M.O. Amdur (Eds.), *Casarett and Doull's Toxicology: The Basic Science of Poisons* 2nd ed. New York: Macmillan Publishers, pp. 468-496.

Hatsukami, D., Owen, P, Pyle, R., & Mitchell, J. (1983). Similarities and differences in the MMPI between women with bulimia and women with alcohol or drug abuse problems. *Addictive Behaviors, 7,* 435-439.

Hechtman, L, Weiss, G., & Perlman, T. (1980). Hyperactives as young adults. *Canadian Journal of Psychiatry, 25,* 4782D482.

Herman, B.E. (1980). A sensory-integrative approach to the psychotic child. *Occupational Therapy in Mental Health, 1*(:1), 57-68.

Herzog, D.B. (1982). Bulimia: The secretive syndrome. *Psychosomatics, 23,* 481-487.

Herzog, D.B., Keller, M.B., & Lavori, P.W. (1988). Outcome in anorexia nervosa and bulimia nervosa: A review of the literature. *Journal of Nervous and Mental Diseases, 176,* 131-143.

Herzog, D.G. (1988). Eating disorders. In A.M. Nicholi (Ed.), *The New Harvard Guide to Psychiatry.* Cambridge, MA: Belknap Press, pp. 434-445.

Hsu, L.K., Crisp, A.H., & Harding, B. (1979). Outcome of anorexia nervosa. *The Lancet, Jan. 13,* 61-65.

Jellinek, M.S. & Herzog, D.B. (1988). The child. In A.M. Nicholi (Ed.), *The New Harvard Guide to Psychiatry.* Cambridge, MA: Belknap Press, pp. 607-636.

Kaye, W.H., Ebert, M.H., Gwirtsman, H.E., & Weiss, S.R. (1984). Differences in brain serotonergic metabolism between nonbulimic and bulimic patients with anorexia nervosa. *American Journal of Psychiatry, 141,* 1598-1601.

Kaye, W.H., Gwirtsman, H.E., George, D.T., Weiss, S.R., & Jimerson, D.C. (1986). Relationship of mood alterations to bingeing behavior in bulimia. *British Journal of Psychiatry, 149,* 479-485.

Kendall, P.C. & Finch, A.J. (1978). A cognitive-behavioral treatment for impulsivity: A group comparison study. *Journal of Consulting and Clinical Psychology, 46,* 110-118.

Kwako, R. (1980). Relaxation as therapy for hyperactive children. *Occupational Therapy in Mental Health, 1*(:3), 29-45.

Love, A.J. & Thompson, M.G.G. (1988). Language disorders and attention deficit disorders in young children referred for psychiatric services: Analysis of prevalence and a conceptual synthesis. *American Journal of Orthopsychiatry, 58,* 52-64.

McCall, M.A., Friedland, J., & Kerr, A. (1986). When doing is not enough: The relationship between activity and effectiveness in anorexia nervosa. *Occupational Therapy in Mental Health, 6*(:1), 137-152.

McEvoy, M.A., Nordquist, V.M., Twardosz, S., Heckaman, K.A., Wehby, J.H., & Denny, R.K. (1988). Promoting autistic children's peer interaction in an integrated early childhood setting using affection activities. *Journal of Applied Behavioral Analysis, 21,* 193-200.

Martin, M.J. (1989). Children with mental retardation. In P.N. Pratt & A.S. Allen, (Eds.), *Occupational Therapy for Children*, 2nd ed. pp. 422-441.

Matson, J.L. (1981). Use of independence training to teach shopping skills to mildly retarded adults. *American Journal of Mental Deficiency, 86,* 178-183.

Minuchin, S., Roseman, B.L., & Baker, L. (1978). *Psychosomatic Families: Anorexia Nervosa in Context.* Cambridge, MA: Harvard University Press.

Morgan, H.G. & Russell, G.F.M. (1975). Value of family background and clincial features as predictors of long-term outcome in anorexia nervosa: Four-year follow-up study of 41 patients. *Psychological Medicine, 5,* 355-371.

Nelson, D.L. (1981). Evaluating autistic clients. *Occupational Therapy in Mental Health, 1*(4), 1-22.

Nicholi, A.M. Jr. (1988). The adolescent. In A.M. Nicholi (Ed.), *The New Harvard Guide to Psychiatry.* Cambridge, MA: Belknap Press, pp. 637-664.

Norman, D.K. & Herzog, D.B. (1984). Persistent social maladjustment in bulimia: A 1-year follow-up. *American Journal of Psychiatry, 141,* 444-446.

Offer, D., Marcus, D., Offer, J.L. (1970). A longitudinal study of normal adolescent boys. *American Journal of Psychiatry, 126,* 917-924.

Patterson, G.R. (1979). Treatment for children with conduct problems: A review of outcome studies. In S. Feshback & A. Fraczek (Eds.), *Aggression and Behavior Change: Biological and Social Process.* New York: Praeger.

Pope, H.G., Hudson, J.L., & Yurgelun-Todd, D. (1984). Anorexia nervosa and bulimia among 300 women shoppers. *American Journal of Psychiatry, 141,* 292-294.

Pope, H.S., Hudson, J.L., Jonas, T.M., Yurgelun-Todd, D. (1985). Antidepressant treatment of bulemia: A 2-year follow-up study. *Journal of Clinical Psychopharmacology, 5,* 320-327.

Robins, L.N. (1970). The adult development of the antisocial child. *Seminars in Psychiatry, 2,* 420-434.

Robins, L.N. (1978). Sturdy childhood predictors of adult antisocial behaviors: Replication from longitudinal studies. *Psychology & Medicine, 8,* 611-622.

Robinson, P.W., Newby, T.J., & Ganzell, S.L. (1981). A token system for a class of underachieving hyperactive children. *Journal of Applied Behavioral Analysis, 14,* 192-198.

Roff, J.D. & Wirt, R.D. (1984). Childhood social adjustment, adolescent status, and young adult mental health. *American Journal of Orthopsychiatry, 54,* 595-602.

Rumsey, J.M., Rapoport, J.L., & Sceery, W.R. (1985). Autistic children as adults: Psychiatric, social and behavioral outcomes. *Journal of the American Academy of Child Psychiatry, 24,* 465-473.

Rutter, M. & Taylor, E. (1978). Hyperkinetic disorders in psychiatric clinic attendrs. *Developmental Medicine and Child Neurology, 20,* 279-299.

Rutter, M., & Hersov. L. (Eds.): (1985). *Child Psychiatry: Modern Approaches* 2nd ed. London: Blackwell Scientific Publishing.

Satterfield, J.H., Satterfield, B.T., & Cantwell, D.P. (1981). Three-year multimodality treatment study of 100 hyperactive boys. *Behavioral Pediatrics, 98,* 650-655.

Schalock, R.L., Harper, R.S., & Carver, G. (1981). Independent living placement: Five years later. *American Journal of Mental Deficiency, 2,* 170-177.

Schwartz, R., Barrett, M.J., & Saba, G. (1985). Family therapy for bulimia. In D.M. Garner & P.E. Garfinkel (Eds.), *Handbook of Psychotherapy for Anorexia Nervosa and Bulimia.* New York: Guilford Press.

Shah, A. & Holmes, N. (1987). Locally-based residential services for mentally handicapped adults: A comparative study. *Psychological Medicine, 17,* 763-774.

Stoner, S.B. & Glynn, M.A. (1987). Cognitive styles of school-age children showing attention deficit disorders with hyperactivity. *Psychological Reports, 61,* 119-125.

Ward, A.J. (1978). Early childhood autism and structrual therapy: Outcome after 3 years. *Journal of Consulting and Clinical Psychology, 46,* 1978.

Zimmerman, I.L. & Woo-Sam, J.M. (1984). Intellectual assessment of children. In G. Goldstein & M. Hersen (Eds.), *Handbook of Psychological Assessment.* New York: Pergamon Press, pp. 57-76.

Chapter 4
Organic Mental Disorders and Syndromes

This category of DSM-III-R diagnoses includes those that are associated with known or suspected biological etiologies and characterized by brain dysfunction. There are two major categories: syndromes, a label for constellations of symptoms that reflect brain dysfunction where the specific source of the dysfunction is not identified; and disorders, where an Axis III diagnosis coexists, i.e., a specific disease entity or causative agent has been identified. This distinction is imprecise, as not all disorders have well-understood disease processes. It is fairly common for an individual first entering treatment to be diagnosed with a syndrome, as the precise agent causing the cognitive disorder may not be readily apparent. After further testing, the source of the problem, a specific drug or disease, for example, may become clear and the diagnosis may be changed to a disorder.

Organic Mental Disorders and Syndromes are all marked by changes in cognition, with accompanying mood changes, anxiety, or changes in self-esteem and personality. The cognitive alterations are a defining characteristic of organic brain disorders. It should be noted that this diagnostic group has undergone considerable change as understanding of biological/neurological processes has increased. Very broad categories such as "organic brain syndrome," which appeared in earlier diagnostic lists, have been replaced with much more specific and precise diagnoses.

Organic Mental Syndromes

The main diagnoses in this category are dementia, delirium, intoxication, withdrawal, and several function-specific categories (e.g., organic anxiety syndrome, organic mood syndrome). They describe states and behaviors, rather than causes, though by definition a physiological cause is implied. For example, intoxication requires ingestion of some psychoactive substance, but the syndrome, unlike the disorder, does not specify what substance. Dementia and delirium will be discussed together to clarify the similarities and differences between the two conditions. This will be followed by separate discussions of intoxication and of other organic mental syndromes. Discussion of withdrawal will be deferred to the next chapter, where substance abuse is considered.

Figure 4-1
Organic Mental Syndromes & Disorders

Organic Mental Syndromes	Organic Mental Disorders

Dementia
    cognitive change
    full consciousness
	Dementias arising in the senium &
	    presenium

Delirium
    cognitive change
    altered consciousness
Intoxication
Withdrawal
	Psychoactive substance
	    induced mental disorders

Delirium and Dementia

Both delirium and dementia are characterized by global changes in cognition. The difference between the two is the level of consciousness of the individual. (See Fig. 4-1) In the case of delirium, consciousness is diminished, whereas in dementia the individual will be fully conscious. In addition to altered consciousness, delirium presents with inability to maintain attention, disorganized thinking, changes in psychomotor activity or sleep, disorientation, and memory impairment. Onset is generally rapid, and a precipitating event can frequently be identified. Occasionally, the diagnosis is made in the absence of organic findings if the symptoms cannot be attributed to some other disorder. Seltzer (1988) defines delirium as a clouding of consciousness with global cognitive impairment and disorientation. Onset is usually sudden and associated with an obvious disease process such as hypoxia, hypoglycemia, an endocrine disorder, neurological disorder, intoxication, etc. For example, a child with a high fever may seem "out of it," be confused, or hard to rouse.

Dementia is characterized by memory loss in the presence of full consciousness. Abstract thinking and judgment may be impaired, aphasia, apraxia, and other cognitive and motor disabilities may be noted along with personality changes, such as newly developing paranoia. For the diagnosis to be made, symptoms must be sufficiently severe to interfere with vocational or social functioning. As indicated above, changes in consciousness are not noted. An individual with this syndrome would appear fully alert but might not recognize family members, might not be oriented to time or place, and so on. The diagnosis is made in the presence of symptoms if a biological cause is presumed. Once a specific cause has been identified, such as Pick's or Alzheimer's disease, the diagnosis will be changed to disorder.

Etiology and Incidence

By definition, these syndromes are presumed to have biological causes. Delirium may accompany a high fever, head trauma, or many other physical problems. In the case of dementia, differential diagnosis on Axis III is critical, as the cause of dementia defines treatment. Thus, in most instances, the syndrome diagnosis is temporary until the precise nature of the problem can be identified. Some "pseudodementias" may be hysterical or depressive in etiology. Although depression in older adults may initially present with symptoms of dementia, it is treated much differently from Alzheimer's disease or multi-infarct dementia and must be ruled out as diagnosing a dementing disorder. There are a large number of causes for dementia, as will be described in the disorder section below. They include such diseases as Alzheimer's disease, Pick's disease, Jakob-Creutzfeldt disease, Huntington's chorea, encephalitis, and diseases related to human immunodeficiency virus (e.g., acquired immune deficiency syndrome). A variety of toxic substances may cause dementia, as will some brain trauma and vascular disease. When a specific cause can be identified, a diagnosis of disorder will be applied.

Both delirium and dementia are extremely common in both men and women, and numbers of dementia cases are increasing, as many dementing illnesses appear in older adults and this population is growing rapidly. In cases that occur later in life, dementia is more frequent in women.

Prognosis

Prognosis is very much dependent on specific etiology; thus it is harder to predict outcomes for syndromes, where the specific cause is not known, as opposed to disorders, in which the cause has been identified. Further discussion of prognosis will be included in the section on disorders, below.

Implications for Function and Treatment

By definition, all these syndromes have a major impact on function. These diagnoses are not made until vocational functioning is impaired. Function in leisure and self-care is also severely compromised. In delirium, onset is rapid; in dementia it is slower and more progressive. The changes that occur are clearly at the skill level, with cognition most obviously and profoundly affected. Motor, sensory, sensorimotor, psychological, and social skills are also affected either immediately or over the course of the disease. Individuals are unable to accurately interpret incoming sensory input: visual, tactile, auditory, kinesthetic, or olfactory. They have difficulty performing motor skills such as reading, writing, and dressing, both because of difficulty interpreting input and difficulty controlling motor output. Because skills are so impaired, performance of ADL/IADL, work and leisure activities is also severely impaired.

As dementia progresses, ataxia, apraxia, and other sensorimotor deficits may begin to accompany the earlier cognitive losses. Vocational and leisure performance are affected almost immediately as ability to read, write, and perform in unfamiliar situations are compromised. Later, IADL and ADL abilities will be impaired. The impairment may appear first as an inability to remember to do something, later as an inability to perform the activity. In delirium, all these deficits are likely to appear at once.

An interesting feature of most dementias is that social skills, at least superficial forms of social interaction, are preserved until late in the progress of the syndrome. Individuals may be able to manage simple interaction for some time, and, in fact, may mask much severe cognitive impairments in doing so. Individuals with delirium are unlikely to retain social skills.

Discussion of intervention can be found below, in the section on disorders.

Intoxication

This group of syndromes is characterized by constellations of organic symptoms as the result of substance ingestion. It is differentiated from substance abuse disorders (which are discussed in the following chapter). These are syndromes associated with specific episodes of substance ingestion, whereas substance abuse is a more probable diagnosis where a pattern of continuing abuse has emerged. In addition, substance abuse may or may not result in one of these syndromes. The diagnosis is made when there is evidence of recent ingestion of a psychoactive substance and there are changes in consciousness, mood, attentiveness, motor function, with impaired judgment, social, or vocational functioning.

Etiology and Incidence

By definition, etiology is the ingestion of a psychoactive substance. When a diagnosis of syndrome is made, the specific substance has not been identified.

These syndromes are quite common in both males and females.

Prognosis

In most cases, prognosis for the immediate episode is good, with function restored as the substance is excreted from the system. Intoxication may last from a few hours to several days, but is almost always self-limiting, unlike the substance abuse disorders. This kind of abuse is common among college students, for example, where substances may be ingested periodically without a pattern of abuse emerging. For some, one episode of intoxication is enough to prevent further abuse. There are some exceptions to this rule as, for example, with LSD, which has been described as causing "flashbacks" in some individuals.

It is possible in some instances for death to occur as a result of excessive ingestion. These deaths are occasionally the result of fraternity "hazing," for instance, where new members are encouraged to drink alcohol to excess. It is also possible for death to occur as a result of behaviors in which the individual engages while intoxicated, notably, but not limited to, automobile accidents.

Implications for Function and Treatment

During these acute episodes, function is generally significantly impaired in occupational, social, and self-care spheres. This dysfunction is the result of cognitive impairment, with accompanying distortion of sensation, motor skill, and judgment. As the intoxicating substance is eliminated, function returns to normal. "Normal" in many of these individuals represents an impaired level of function as the result of an ongoing substance abuse disorder.

Treatment involves preventing further ingestion of substance, and management of symptoms while the system clears of the substance. In some cases, for instance, seizures may occur and must be managed.

Other Organic Syndromes

There are several other organic syndromes that are characterized by less global impairment. These include amnestic syndrome, hallucinosis, delusional syndrome, mood syndrome, organic syndrome, and personality syndrome. The name of each suggests the specific area in which symptoms appear. For example, organic mood syndrome is characterized by changes in mood as the result of organic factors, organic personality syndrome, personality changes, and so on. If symptoms of delirium or dementia are also present, the more global diagnosis will be made.

Etiology and Incidence

A variety of physical problems may result in these syndromes. Included among them are tumors, metabolic or endocrine disorders, and exposure to toxic substances. As with other syndromes, once the specific etiological agent is identified, the diagnosis will change to disorder. As with other organic mental syndromes, these are quite common in both men and women.

Prognosis

In each case, prognosis is dependent on cause, with some of the metabolic and endocrine disorders, for example, being treatable medically whereas some tumors are not. Some toxicities are reversible, others are not. It is only once the diagnosis can be shifted to disorder that it is possible to determine prognosis.

Implications for Function and Treatment

By definition, functional impairment caused by these disorders is limited, often to a particular sphere. In organic amnestic syndrome, for example, memory is affected but other function is not. Thus, these individuals can manage ADL and most IADL, and continue to function socially (although they may not remember significant others). Vocational function is dependent on the particular memory impairment, but may be intact. Memory for the specific work environment may be affected, however, so that the individual can remember how to program a computer, but possibly not the specific computer programming job on which he or she was working.

Treatment can be implemented only once a cause has been identified, so early intervention focuses on determining the etiology.

Organic Mental Disorders

This group of diagnoses, unlike organic syndromes, is characterized by relationship to a specific, known organic disease, or to ingestion of a specific substance. Thus, when an Axis III diagnosis can be made, i.e., the particular cause of the symptoms is known, an organic disorder diagnosis is more likely to be made.

Dementias Arising in the Senium and Presenium

This diagnosis is becoming increasingly common and the numbers will continue to increase as the population ages (Goldman, 1984). It is not clear at this point that there is a difference between early (presenile) and later (senile) onset dementias, although some clinicians continue to believe that they have different characteristics. It is clear, however, that these disorders are not what was once referred to as senility. Nor do they represent benign senescent forgetfulness (Kral, 1978), the sort of minor memory change characteristic of normal aging but is *not* disabling. A standard example is that forgetting where you put your glasses is a sign of benign senescent forgetfulness; forgetting you wear glasses may be a sign of dementia.

This group of diagnoses includes the dementias that appear most often (although not exclusively) in older individuals. There is a large number of possible causes of dementia, and the identification of a cause is necessary to diagnosis of a disorder as opposed to a syndrome. Causes include Alzheimer's disease, vascular disease (multi-infarct dementia), Huntington's chorea, Pick's disease, Jakob-Creutzfeldt and multiple-sclerosis. There are other, reversible causes of dementia, including depression, and metabolic and nutritional problems, and there is a group of dementias labeled pseudodementia (e.g., Ganser's syndrome) that are thought to be psychogenic rather than biological in origin. Ganser's syndrome is more likely to occur in younger individuals in stressful situations (Seltzer, 1988). Differential diagnosis is somewhat difficult at present, but vital to effective treatment. By far the most common dementing illness is dementia of the Alzheimer's type (DAT) or Alzheimer's disease. It is believed to account for at least half of dementias in the elderly.

Distinguishing among the dementias is done on the basis of both laboratory findings and the nature of the symptoms. DAT and Pick's are primarily coritcal, whereas Huntington's and Parkinson's diseases are subcortical (Cummings, 1982). Multi-infarct and Jakob-Creutzfeldt are mixed. The subcoritcal dementias have more extrapyramidal signs, such as ataxia and tremor, whereas the cortical dementias have more cognitive symptoms such as memory loss, personality change and visuospatial impairment. Recognition of these symptom differences is an important step in diagnosis.

Diagnosis of DAT must be made by exclusion. It can be confirmed only through brain biopsy or autopsy. If other causes of dementia, including depression, metabolic orders and multi-infarct dementia, can be ruled out, a diagnosis of DAT will be made. Multi-infarct dementia can be diagnosed by computerized axial tomography (CAT scan), as it is caused by small infarcts in the cerebral vascular system. These two dementias present differing clinical pictures as well. Multi-infarct dementias are characterized by spotty loss of function, which progresses through rather abrupt changes in performance followed by periods of relative stability. The individual might have language problems that are fairly stable until the sudden addition of a personality change. DAT, on the other hand, shows more global loss and more gradual, continuous progression. These differences may be quite subtle, however.

Etiology and Incidence

Multi-infarct dementia is caused by a series of small cerebral vascular tears or infarcts. Each leads to cerebral hypoxia and tissue death in small areas of the brain with accompanying loss of function. The precise etiology of DAT is not known, although autopsy reveals a characteristic pattern of neuritic plaques and tangles (Cummings, 1982). A variety of etiological factors have been hypothesized. The most prevalent theories at present include a genetic explanation, a slow virus (as has been demonstrated in Jakob-Creutzfeldt disease), or some unexplained loss of neurotransmitters.

It appears that there may be more than one type of DAT. A number of researchers have speculated that there is a familial (genetic) form of DAT that differs symptomatically from other forms, as well as having a different etiology (Heston, Mastri, Anderson, & White, 1981; Silverman, Breitner, Mohs, & Davis, 1986). Although this type of Alzheimer's disease has been difficult to document because of diagnostic problems and deaths from unrelated causes, an autosomal dominant familial form has been identified. In affected families, the odds are 50% that children or siblings of the individual will develop the disorder if they live long enough.

A distinction is made between early and late onset dementia (Chui, Teng, Henderson, & Moy, 1985). It appears that early onset dementia is more severe, with worse aphasia (speech difficulty) and presence of agraphia (difficulty writing) early on. Some researchers have speculated that the early onset type is the familial type, but this contention is still open to debate with research both supporting and refuting this supposition.

There has been increasing research about DAT, which has been found to be present in approximately 50% of all nursing home residents (Seltzer, 1988). Since the numbers are likely to increase, considerable attention has been given to the disorder. Other dementias are also increasing. Approximately 5% to 6% of the population over age 65 has some form of dementia and the numbers are increasing rapidly (Berezin, Liptzin, & Salzman, 1988). Probably because of differential life expectancies, the disorders are more common in women.

Prognosis

Prognosis for DAT is always poor. The disease progresses to total incapacity and death. The speed of progress is quite variable, however. Some researchers speculate that early onset DAT is more likely to progress rapidly, to result in greater dysfunction, and to cause death within a few years. By contrast, later onset DAT is thought to progress more slowly, with the possibility of functional plateaus that last for long periods. Different course as a result of age of onset is not clearly established, but it is known that DAT will progress over time and is always fatal.

Prognosis for multi-infarct dementia is variable. Existing damage is irreversible, but the disease may progress slowly, or not at all. Treatment of coexisting high blood pressure or vascular disease may slow or stop the progress of the disease.

The other irreversible dementias also have poor long-term prognoses. The only one with any particularly effective treatment is Parkinson's disease, which can be treated symptomatically with the medication levodopamine (L-dopa). Otherwise, management rather than treatment is the goal of intervention.

Implications for Function and Treatment

These disorders have a devastating impact on all areas of function. As they progress, occupational, social, and ADL/IADL skills disappear, until, ultimately, swallowing and even breathing may become difficult. Death often occurs as a result of pneumonia, which is the result of inability to clear the lungs. As noted above, the progress of the diseases is somewhat variable and rather unpredictable. Some residual function may be retained for long periods. A person might be able to play checkers for many years as other functions diminish, especially if the game was a favorite long-standing occupation.

DAT has been described as progressing through three stages (Cummings, 1982). The first symptom identified is usually memory impairment. The individual may put water on the stove to boil and forget to turn it off, or may go out and forget how to get back home. The memory difficulties may lead to work problems and carelessness in personal grooming. For example, the individual may forget how to do work tasks or forget to bathe. During the second stage, aphasia, apraxia (movement difficulties), disorientation, and restlessness appear. It is common during this phase to see the individual pacing around the house for hours on end, forgetting who people are, even those closest to him or her, having difficulty finding words. In some individuals, an attempt to deal with the word-finding problem is made by talking around the word. Thus, a "radio" may be called "the machine with a switch that talks." The individual may become unable to read or to recognize others. The spouse may find that the affected individual now identifies him or her as a sister or brother or parent rather than as a spouse.

Personality changes also occur. Temper outbursts are common as the individual finds his or her limitations extremely frustrating. In addition, as ability to understand the environment worsens, the individual becomes fearful and often paranoid. When personal items are missing, the individual often assumes that they have been stolen. Finally, memory becomes severely impaired and total loss of sensory and cognitive abilities occurs. The individual becomes bedridden and incontinent, unable to chew or swallow.

Some specific characteristics of the symptoms are worth noting. First, personality and social behavior may be maintained well into the disease. In fact, some individuals learn to cover their impairment so well that it is not recognized by others until the disease is well along. It is only after listening for awhile that the other person becomes aware that verbalizations, however pleasant, make no sense. This can present problems for the individual who wanders off and is found by police. The memory and sensory losses also have some specific characteristics. Problems seem to arise in the encoding of information, so the defect is in recent rather than immediate or remote memory (LaRue, 1982). This means that the individual will be able to process what is happening at the moment and what happened 50 years ago, but not what happened that morning. In addition, extraneous memories seem to intrude on function, leading to confabulation and perseveration. An individual who is questioned about family members may present a long, rambling description of his or her sisters and brothers as children, but not remember spouse and children. This is a characteristic that distinguishes DAT from depression, which is more likely to lead to absence of response.

Language, especially word-finding, is almost universally impaired. Articulation, however, remains intact until very late in the disease course (Murdoch, Chenery, Wilks, & Boyle, 1987). The individual can say "car," but not know what it is, or use that word to form an idea. Aphasia is thought to be worse in the familial type, and agraphia (inability to write) is a defining feature of familial DAT. Visuospatial deficits are common, as are visual field losses (Steffes & Thralow, 1987). The individual thus has difficulty with dressing, walking, and other activities which require spatial discrimination. Temporal distortions are also common (Cummings, 1982), with the person unable to keep track of time, day, or season.

Other dementias are characterized by different functional deficits. Pick's disease, which has an earlier onset than DAT (usually between ages 40 and 60), manifests itself first with behavioral and affective changes (Cummings, 1982). Cognitive changes, including aphasia, occur later. Unlike DAT, motor and sensory changes are rare, and occur later in the disease course. Visuospatial deficits are also rare.

Multi-infarct dementia has less predictable functional consequences, as changes are dependent on the location and extent of cerebral damage (Hachinski, Lassen, & Marshall, 1974). In addition, progress of the disease is inconsistent. There may be long periods of plateau and sudden decrements in performance.

Careful identification of both the course and the symptoms of dementia is, as has been noted, crucial. The pseudodementias, in particular, present with a different course, and are more likely to be treatable or reversible (McAllister, 1983). Although there is some disagreement about what constitutes a pseudodementia, it seems that there are at least two categories: depressive dementias and hysterical dementias. Depressive dementias are a manifestation of depression most likely to appear in the elderly. Instead of symptoms of sadness and hopelessness, the depression presents with confusion and memory impairment. Unlike the dementias described above, however, motor slowing and reduced levels of response to the environment are seen. This type of dementia is reversible through drug therapy. Hysterical dementias are those that have no identifiable biological base, and seem to be the result of psychological conflict and stress rather than biology. They are usually identifiable by the course, which is atypical for any of the known dementias, and by the fact that the dementia may come and go, with periods of normal function interspersed with problem behavior. Usual treatment for these dementias is psychotherapy and possibly drug therapy.

There are, of course, other causes of dementia, including Korsakoff's disease, Wernicke's encephalopathy and syphillitic dementia. Korsakoff's disease and Wernicke's encephalopathy are attributable to long-term alcoholism; syphillitic dementia, to tertiary syphillis. Wernicke's disease can be treated; the other two are irreversible, although they may stabilize rather than progress. Each has its own particular course and symptoms. Korsakoff's disease, for example, presents with amnesia for recent events. The individual remembers quite clearly up to a point, perhaps 10 years ago, and has no memory for anything that occurred from that time to the present. Wernicke's encephalopathy has symptoms more typical of delirium, and, in addition, signs of brain-stem damage such as eye-movement paralysis (Seltzer, 1988).

A new dementia emerging in rapidly growing numbers is that related to acquired immune deficiency syndrome (AIDS). It appears that as many as two-thirds of AIDS victims have some degree of dementia (Navia, Jordan & Price, 1986). In fact, it has been speculated that some early features of dementia, including subtle neurological and personality changes, may occur as a precursor to the symptoms of AIDS in individuals infected with the human immunodeficiency virus.

AIDS dementia complex has many of the features of other dementias, but progresses very rapidly. It is separate from some of the opportunistic infections that cause encephalitis or other CNS diseases. Its manifestations are global cognitive impairment, including memory deficits, intellectual impairment, and poor concentration and memory. According to Navia and colleagues (1986), inflicted individuals maintain the ability to do simple ADL, but are not functionally independent. Social, leisure and vocational performance are severely compromised. Late stage individuals are severely dysfunctional in all spheres.

Available treatment of individuals with dementing illness is minimal, except in those cases where a reversible cause can be identified. In the majority of cases, however, treatment is symptomatic and behavioral. If the individual is wandering at night, for example, a low dose of a sleeping medication may be administered. In cases where severe paranoia appears, medication may also be tried. Medical intervention presents problems, though, as drugs may make symptoms worse. Some symptoms can be reasonably well-managed for some time. The most common dementias, however, cannot be cured, nor can the progression be stopped or, in most cases, even slowed. Much intervention focuses on the individual's caregiver, who must learn how to manage the behaviors. The caregiver may be taught how to give simple instructions, how to deal with temper outbursts, and so on (Mace & Robins, 1987).

Implications for Occupational Therapy

Occupational therapists have a vital role to play in the treatment of dementing illnesses. Because of the incurable and usually progressive nature of the disorders, interventions that focus on management and maximizing quality of life are quite valuable. Assessment should include evaluation of the skills of the individual, as well as the circumstances of the family (Bonder, 1986).

In the early stages of these disorders, efforts can be made to help the individual maintain function. This may be done through environmental adaptation, education, and use of assistive devices, particularly memory aids. Exercise may help maintain physical function (Killeffer, Bennett, & Gruen, 1984).

As the individual's function declines, focus shifts to helping caregivers cope with emerging deficits. Again, environmental adaptation can be useful. This includes simplifying the environment, reducing the number of stimuli, and also adding various safety devices, such as automatic turn-off switches for stoves and door alarms to warn of wandering. The caregiver must be educated about the course of the disease and given information about how to deal with problems. It may be helpful to provide information about how to feed the person, how to modify clothing, and so on.

For both the individual and the caregiver, quality of life is a major issue. For the individual, activity should be encouraged at whatever level he or she can perform. Day treatment programs provide structured activities and stimulation at a level that the individual can manage. The caregiver is often overwhelmed and exhausted by the needs of the individual and must be encouraged to take time for his or her own leisure. At some point, nursing home placement may be necessary, and the occupational therapist may join with others involved in care to help the caregiver make this decision.

Following nursing home placement, maintenance of function and enhancement of quality of life continue to be important (Killeffer et al, 1984). Activity should continue at the maximum level possible and families should be active participants in care (Bonder, Miller, & Linsk, unpublished manuscript).

Psychoactive Substance-Induced Organic Mental Disorders

A long list of substances is included in this category, including alcohol, amphetamines, caffeine, cannabis, cocaine, hallucinogens, inhalants, nicotine, opiates, phencyclidine (PCP), and sedatives. As with dementias, the distinction between syndrome and disorder relates to the specificity of the etiology. Disorders of intoxication and withdrawal are known for a wide range of substances. These disorders will not be discussed in detail here, as they are most often acute disorders in which the occupational therapist has little involvement. They are however, common diagnoses in inpatient settings, particularly those that focus on substance abuse. Further discussion of substance abuse, which frequently coexists with substance-induced organic syndromes/disorders, can be found in the next chapter.

When a diagnosis of substance-induced organic mental disorder is made, the same symptoms discussed in sections above are present. The individual may demonstrate delirium, dementia, or any of the more specific organic syndromes. However, they occur in the presence of recent ingestion of a psychoactive substance. Thus, the origin of the problem can be readily identified. In most instances, once withdrawal from the substance is complete, the symptoms disappear. Some of these substances, PCP, for instance, have long-acting effects, meaning that the individual may demonstrate symptoms for relatively long periods following ingestion. Others, especially LSD, appear to cause "flashbacks." For most of these substances, organic mental disorders will not occur unless the individual has a history of abuse. Some substances, like the hallucinogens, may cause symptoms on first exposure. Chronic substance abuse may also cause specific types of dementia. An example is Korsakoff's disease, a long-term consequence of alcohol abuse. It causes permanent retrograde amnesia (Albert, Butters, & Levin, 1979), i.e., the individual lacks memory of events beyond some earlier point in life.

Treatment is usually medical and largely symptomatic, as eventual excretion of the substance will resolve the immediate problem. In cases where the symptoms continue, the occupational therapist may be brought into treatment. These situations are discussed in greater detail in the next chapter. (See Fig. 4-2)

Figure 4-2
Indications of Organic Mental Syndromes and Disorders

Disorder	Symptoms	Functional Deficits
A. Syndromes Delirium	1. Reduced attention	Global ADL/IADL, work, leisure

Figure 4-2 *continued*
Indications of Organic Mental Syndromes and Disorders

Disorder	Symptoms	Functional Deficits
A. Syndromes (cont.) Delirium	2. Disorganized thinking 3. Altered consciousness 4. Rapid onset	Global motor, sensory motor, cognitive, social psychological
Dementia	1. Memory impairment	Global ADL/IADL, work, leisure
	2. Cognitive impairment	Global sensory, sensory motor, cognitive, social, psychological
	3. 1 & 2 interfere with function	May be mild to severe
	4. No altered consciousness	
Intoxication	1. Evidence of recent ingestion of a psychoactive substance	Social, work, leisure
	2. Substance causes maladaptive behavior	Possibly sensory, motor, sensory motor, cognitive, psychological
Withdrawal	1. Symptoms of organic disorder as a result of substance withdrawal	May affect any area
B. Disorders Dementia of the Alzheimer's type	1. Dementia 2. Insidious onset 3. Deteriorating course	Global & progressive
Multi-infarct Dementia	1. Dementia 2. Step-wise, deteriorating ability	Unpredictable & patchy with stable periods

Figure 4-2 *continued*
Organic Mental Syndromes and Disorders

Disorder	Symptoms	Functional Deficits
	3. Laboratory evidence of cerebrovascular disease	

References

Albert, M.S., Butters, N., & Levin, J. (1979). Temporal gradients in the retrograde amnesia of patients with alcoholic Korsakoff's disease. *Archives of Neurology, 36,* 211-216.

Berezin, M.A., Liptzin, B., & Salzman, C. (1988). The elderly person. In A.M. Nieholi (Ed.), *The New Harvard Guide to Psychiatry.* Cambridge, MA: Belknap Press, pp. 665-680.

Bonder, B.R., Miller, B.M., & Linsk, N. Who should do what? Perceptions of staff and caregiver responsibilities for nursing home residents. Unpublished manuscript.

Bonder, B.R. (1986). Family systems and Alzheimer's disease: An approach to treatment. *Physical and Occupational Therapy in Geriatrics, 5*(:2), 13-24.

Chui, H.C., Teng, E.L., Henderson, V.W., & Moy, A.C. (1985). Clinical subtypes of dementia of the Alzheimer type. *Neurology, 35,* 1544-1550.

Cummings, J.I. (1982). Cortical dementias. In D.F. Benson, & D. Blume (Eds.), *Psychiatric Aspects of Neurologic Disease,*Vol. 2. New York: Grune and Stratton, pp. 93-121.

Goldman, R. (1984). The epidemiology and demography of dementia. *Psychiatric Annals, 14,* 169-174.

Hachinski, V.C., Lassen, N.A., & Marshall, J. (1974). Multi-infarct dementia: A cause of mental deterioration in the elderly. *The Lancet, July 27.*

Heston, L.L., Mastri, A.R., Anderson, V.E., & White, J. (1981). Dementia of the Alzheimer type. *Archives of General Psychiatry, 38,* 1085-1090.

Killeffer, A.H.P., Bennett, R., & Gruen, G. (1984). Handbook of innovative programs for the impaired elderly. *Physical and Occupational Therapy in Geriatrics* (special issue). New York: Haworth Press.

Kral, V.A. (1978). Benign senescent forgetfulness. In R. Katzman, R.D. Terry, & K.L. Bick (Eds.), *Alzheimer's Disease: Senile Dementia and Related Disorders.* New York: Raven Press.

LaRue, A. (1982). Memory loss and aging. *Psychiatric Clinics of North America, 5,* 89-103.

McAllister, T.W. (1983). Overview: Pseudodementia. *American Journal of Psychiatry, 140*, 528-533.

Mace, N.L. & Robins, P.V. (1981). *36-Hour Day*. Baltimore: Johns Hopkins University Press.

Murdoch, B.E., Chenery, H.J., Wilks, V., & Boyle, R.S. (1987). Language in Alzheimer dementia. *Brain and Language, 31*, 122-137.

Nevia, B.A., Jordan, B.D., & Price, R.W. (1986). The AIDS dementia complex: I. Clinical features. *Annals of Neurology, 19*, 517-524.

Seltzer, B. (1988). Organic mental disorders. In A.M. Nicholi (Ed.), *The New Harvard Guide to Psychiatry*. Cambridge, MA: Belknap Press, pp. 358-386.

Silverman, J.M., Breitner, J.C.S., Mohs, R.C., & Davis, K.L. (1986). Reliability of the family history method in genetic studies of Alzheimer's disease and related dementias. *American Journal of Psychiatry, 143*, 1279-1282.

Steffes, R., & Thralow, J. (1987). Visual field limitation in the patient with dementia of the Alzheimer's type. *Journal of the American Geriatric Society, 35*, 198-204.

Chapter 5

Psychoactive Substance Use Disorders

In our society, a vast number of substances are abused. Some are considered illicit, among them cannabis, cocaine, PCP, hallucinogens, and opiates. Others are available as prescription medications, useful for specific purposes, but hazardous if misused. This group includes such medications as sedatives. Still other substances are intended for other purposes. Inhalants, for example, include glues, paints, and solvents. One of the most commonly abused substances is alcohol, which is legal, widely available, and socially accepted under many circumstances. Similarly, nicotine is a legal and readily available psychoactive substance with potentially devastating health effects. The illegal substances have been recognized as problematic for years, while disapproval of alcohol and nicotine abuse has been growing only recently. (In the case of alcohol, this represents a return to awareness of the problems of abuse.)

DSM-III-R has two general categories that may apply regardless of the substance being abused, or in cases where several are abused simultaneously. These categories include dependence and abuse (See Fig. 5-1). Each substance is then categorized separately, with characteristics specific to the substance described in more detail.

Dependence is diagnosed when at least three of the following conditions are present: the substance is taken in larger amounts or over more time than the individual planned; efforts to cut down are unsuccessful; and much of the person's activity revolves around getting the substance and other activities are reduced as a result. Obligations are not met, and dangerous behavior may result from intoxication. For example, the individual may miss work, spend paychecks to obtain the substance rather than food, and may drive while intoxicated or begin to steal to have money to pay for the substance. The individual is aware that the problem exists, but develops a tolerance for the substance (i.e., increasing amounts are needed to obtain an effect). In addition, for most of these substances, withdrawal symptoms occur and the individual may take the substance to avoid these symptoms. Thus, even though the individual knows the he or she has a problem, withdrawal becomes so unpleasant that the individual expends considerable effort to continue the substance. Dependence is also characterized by at least 1 month of disturbance. Some earlier descriptions of substance abuse sought to distinguish between dependence and addiction. Dependence was described as a psychological phenomenon, whereas addiction represented a physical need for the substance which led to physical withdrawal symptoms. It has become clear that this is a difficult, and probably arbitrary, distinction and it is no longer made.

Abuse, on the other hand, may be diagnosed when the criteria for dependence are not met, but the individual has noticeable behavioral problems related to psychoactive substance use. The symptoms must be present for at least 1 month, but may not be as global or persistent as those for dependence. An individual might occasionally drink too much, and skip work to gamble at the race track when intoxicated.

Several classes of psychoactive substances have been identified on the basis of similarity of effects. They are alcohol and sedatives, cocaine and amphetamines, hallucinogens and phencyclidine (PCP), inhalants, opioids, cannabis, and nicotine (which is characterized by dependence, but not abuse). Those with similar characteristics will be discussed together. The types of substance abuse most likely to come to the attention of the occupational therapist are described in detail, those less common to occupational therapy clinics are discussed more briefly. Implications for occupational therapy intervention are summarized at the end of the chapter.

Figure 5-1
Psychoactive Substance Abuse

- alcohol & sedatives
- cocaine & amphetamines
- hallucinogens & phencyclidines
- inhalants
- opioids
- cannabis
- nicotine

Alcohol and Sedatives

Both these groups of substances are CNS depressants. Although alcohol may cause a brief sense of excitement, both alcohol and sedatives slow responses over time. The "high" that accompanies them is actually a slowing of CNS as well as autonomic function. In cases of overdose, death may occur as a result of respiratory or cardiac slowing.

Alcohol use and abuse are common in the United States, although many people in this country either refrain from its use or drink little. Among heavy drinkers, three main patterns of abuse appear. One is characterized by daily intake of large amounts of alcohol, the second by regular binges, on weekends, for example. The third pattern is characterized by long periods of abstinence interspersed with heavy binges. Any of these patterns may occur in alcoholism, although alcoholics who do not drink on a daily basis often point to this as evidence that they have no problem. Other substance abuse, particularly for nicotine, is frequently present in these individuals. So-called "polydrug" abuse is a significant problem (Vaillant, 1988).

Sedatives include barbiturates ("reds," "downers," "yellow jackets") and benzodiazepines (such as valium and librium). Sedatives are characterized by two common patterns of abuse. In some individuals, the drug may be prescribed for a specific purpose, but tolerance may develop and symptoms of dependence appear. Cases in which these drugs are prescribed for long periods to allow an individual to function, as in severe anxiety, do not qualify as substance abuse. In cases of abuse, however, obtaining the drug becomes a primary concern and function changes in negative ways as a result. The second pattern of abuse is seen in individuals who obtain the drug through illicit means, specifically for purposes of abuse, ie, for the "high." In both cases, tolerance is marked.

Etiology and Incidence

There are several theories about the emergence of alcoholism. A familial pattern, evident even when children are raised by adoptive parents, suggests a genetic component in at least some cases (Goodwin, 1984). Goodwin (1984) suggests that familial and non-familial alcoholism may be two different diseases. During the early part of the century, the pre-prohibition and prohibition years, alcoholism was thought to be a moral failure. Since that time, it has come to be viewed as a disease, and that is now the commonly held explanation. Although the origins of alcoholism are not entirely clear, individual and racial differences in alcohol tolerance, separate from dependence and abuse, have been noted. For example, individuals of Oriental origin are much more likely to have severe reactions to alcohol than Caucasians, and therefore to drink less. As with other forms of substance abuse, alcoholism is more common in individuals with personality disorders (Grinspoon & Bakalar, 1988). In addition, alcoholics appear more likely to be suicidal (Berglund, 1983).

Alcohol abuse is of particular importance in adolescents as there is a substantial body of evidence suggesting that it is the first substance abused by almost all adolescents who go on to abuse other drugs (Kandel & Faust, 1975; Yamaguchi & Kandel, 1984). Although this does not mean alcohol abuse causes other substance abuse or that all adolescents who use alcohol will escalate to other drugs, it may be an important prognostic sign and provide a clue that prevention and intervention efforts may be needed.

Dependence on sedatives is less well explained. For individuals who are exposed to the drugs as a result of some other condition, dependence probably results from the effects of the drug itself. Among those who experiment with sedatives as illicit drugs, personality disorders that may predispose to drug experimentation, e.g., antisocial personality, may be precursors of the problem.

Approximately 13% of the adult population of the United States has had problems with alcohol dependence at some point during their lives (APA, 1987). The incidence of sedative dependence is roughly 1.1% of the population (APA, 1987).

Prognosis

Some individuals simply stop abusing both types of substance. The exact percentage of spontaneous remissions is not known. Others benefit from treatment, although some continue abuse throughout their lives, typically lives shortened by the dependence (Vaillant, 1988). It does seem that some alcoholics go on to drink more moderately (Gottheil, Thornton, Skoloda, & Alterman, 1982). This finding is controversial, as the vast majority of treatment programs hold that alcoholics must be totally abstinent to avoid relapse. Without further evidence on the point, the latter view must be taken as accurate.

Follow-up studies suggest that about 50% of alcoholics will continue to have drinking problems while others will be abstinent or controlled drinkers (Polich, Armor, & Braiker, 1980). Gottheil and colleagues (1982) note that individuals may shift between these groups at various times without apparent reasons.

Prognosis for sedative abuse is similarly mixed. One study found that approximately half the abusers continued abuse after treatment (Allgulander, Borg, & Vikander, 1984) and another 30% continued to use the substances. Almost a quarter also abused alcohol.

Alcoholism is a serious problem with major physical consequences. Individuals who continue abuse frequently suffer liver damage and may have signs of organic brain disorders such as Korsakoff's disease, as noted in the previous chapter.

Implications for Function and Treatment

For these diagnoses to be made, functional impairment must be present. Since these substances are all CNS depressants, recent ingestion may lead to drowsiness, reductions in perceptual and motor function, and accompanying problems in ability to perform. Vocational and social performance are most commonly affected, although later stages of dependence, particularly if organic signs appear, may result in decrements in all areas of function. Early in the disease, leisure and social activities are most affected, with the individual's primary leisure and social activity being substance ingestion. As time goes on, family life suffers as the individual spends more time drinking. Work behavior is impaired as the individual either misses time from work as a result of hangovers, or performs poorly because of intoxication on the job.

Of special importance is the likelihood of injury resulting from driving while intoxicated. Industrial accidents may also result from impaired motor and perceptual abilities while under the influence. Withdrawal symptoms may lead the individual to spend a great deal of time obtaining the substance, or to become irritable or enraged. ADL and IADL are rarely severely impaired, although some individuals lose interest in eating as the disorder progresses. Nutritional deficiencies may result from poor diet and may ultimately lead to Wernicke's encephalopathy caused by a B_1 vitamin deficiency. Individuals may become forgetful, resulting in chores undone, checkbooks unbalanced, and so on.

Special note should be made of social role performance. Individuals who are dependent on these substances spend much of their leisure time obtaining and using the substance. They prefer the company of others who are dependent. In addition, if their spouses and family members do not desert them, the family members may feel compelled to hide the abuse, thereby supporting it. This pattern has been described as "codependence" and is problematic in efforts to treat dependence. Individuals themselves may go to great lengths to hide the extent of the problem, for example, drinking before they go to parties or hiding liquor in other containers.

Performance decrements may well be due to CNS changes. It is clear that intoxication causes such alterations (Cohen, Schandler, & Naliboff, 1983). Although the changes diminish to some extent following detoxification, subtle neurological signs may persist and, if abuse continues, become more prominent.

A wide variety of treatments have been attempted, including various milieu and behavioral interventions. One of the best known, and apparently most successful, treatments is Alcoholics Anonymous (AA) (Vaillant, 1988). This is a self-help group that has a philosophy based in a specific set of religious and moral beliefs. Family members may benefit from Al-Anon or Alateen, related groups that address their concerns. AA or other self-help groups may be linked to formal alcoholism treatment programs. Typically for both sedative and alcohol abuse, recognition of the problem and willingness to do something about it are important first steps.

Cocaine and Amphetamines

Unlike alcohol and sedatives, these substances are "uppers," which result in a "high" and psychomotor excitement. Their effects are very similar, though longer lasting with amphetamines. Cocaine may be inhaled, smoked (in the case of the "freebase" or "crack" form) or injected.

Etiology and Incidence

Both substances tend to be abused in similar patterns, two of which are prominent. The first involves daily use of the substance, the second, binges of varying frequency. Amphetamine ("speed") abuse tends to emerge following use of the medications to assist in dieting. Although this use of the drug for this purpose has been largely discredited, some physicians still prescribe it. Cocaine is strictly illicit, although it has been considered trendy by middle and upper class individuals. At the same time, the numbers of lower class individuals abusing cocaine has increased dramatically as crack has become more readily available and cheaper. Both can be highly addictive, with only a few exposures leading to both withdrawal symptoms and increasing desire for the effects. Cocaine abuse has increased dramatically among adolescents (Washton, Gold, Pottash, & Semlitz, 1984).

Of these two dependencies, cocaine is by far the greater concern at present in this country. Estimates of incidence are probably extremely low. Early in the 1980s it was estimated as .2% of the population (APA, 1987), but use has increased dramatically since that time. Crack use in some communities has reached epidemic proportions.

Prognosis

Prognosis for both types of abuse is poor, as the substances are so highly addictive. In addition, until recently, cocaine enjoyed a somewhat glamorous image. Recent deaths of movie stars and athletes as a result of cocaine ingestion has changed that image somewhat. Although those individuals received much attention, the problem is probably worst among poor individuals. The increased availability of crack and reductions in cost have increased the probability that individuals will continue to abuse the drug. Although the pleasurable effects of these substances diminish over time, the craving does not. In addition, abuse of sedatives or alcohol frequently accompanies abuse of these substances to reduce some of the undesirable effects of the drugs such as anxiety and insomnia. Thus, the picture is complicated by addiction to several substances at once. An even more sobering picture is presented by addiction to cocaine and heroin together, a problem that will be discussed further below.

Implications for Function and Treatment

As with alcohol and sedative dependence, abuse of these substances is most likely to affect vocational and social performance. Irritability is pronounced and social withdrawal may develop and become pronounced. Use of the drug becomes the primary avocational interest, thus affecting function in this sphere as well. ADL and IADL are affected as organic (CNS) signs begin to appear, or as need for the drug begins to supersede the wish to attend to these activities.

Some individuals who abuse these drugs turn to criminal activity to support the habit. They may steal or become prostitutes to pay for the drug as their ability to hold jobs decreases and their need for the drug increases. Others become drug pushers themselves.

Treatment is problematic and still poorly developed. AA type interventions may be valuable. Some medical attention may be necessary to prevent complications during withdrawal. In general, however, current efforts to treat these types of abuse are not particularly effective. Several problems have been noted in treatment efforts. First, there is no medication to ameliorate withdrawal effects. Second, unlike some other substances, the pleasurable effect, though diminished over time, continues to occur. Third, there is an increasingly well-developed culture around these drugs, particularly in ghetto environments (Govriti, 1989). Thus, there may be little motivation to withdraw, and little medical help for those who do wish to do so.

Hallucinogens and PCP

Etiology and Incidence

Abuse of these substances appears to be somewhat less than it was 2 decades ago. Initial contact with these substances usually occurs as a result of experimentation with drugs. Personality disorders or adjustment problems are considered to be predisposing factors that might encourage such experimentation. They are often contaminated with or taken with other substances, particularly cannabis and alcohol. PCP ("angel dust," "crystal," "hog") is easily synthesized and may be abused more often than other drugs in this category.

Users find the effects unpredictable. For some individuals, one exposure to the negative effects, particularly during an early experience with the drug, is sufficient to end its use. A "bad trip" may convince a user to stop. Occasionally, a pattern of long term abuse may emerge. Heavier use has been correlated with flashbacks, although the exact nature and cause of this phenomenon is not clear (Naditch & Fenwick, 1977). It may be the result of neurological changes caused by the drug or a hysterical phenomenon.

Prognosis

Most individuals abuse these drugs for relatively short periods before resuming previous activities, although some use them daily for years (Grinspoon & Bakalar, 1988). For most people these drugs prompt experimentation but not usually long term addiction. PCP is the most dangerous, and some individuals seem to develop psychotic disorders as a result of use. For these individuals, the problem is much more intractable.

Implications for Function and Treatment

While the drugs are being abused, performance is severely impaired in all spheres. This is a direct result of the effects of the drugs, which cause hallucinations and cognitive and perceptual dysfunction. It is rare, however, to see such individuals in treatment as a result of dependence or abuse of these two classes of drugs. The exception is when an organic mental disorder appears, as is more likely to be the case with PCP.

Treatment may be warranted if abuse persists. In these cases, principles employed with other forms of substance abuse are likely to be used.

Opioids

Among this group of drugs are some that are clearly illicit, such as heroin and morphine, and others that may be prescribed as analgesics, anesthetics, or cough suppressants. The latter group includes codeine, hydromorphone, methadone, and others. Used in properly supervised medical settings, none of the latter group should lead to dependence, but many of them are used without supervision or are obtained through illicit sources. Methadone is a special problem. Used as a treatment for opioid addiction, it is itself addicting, though it does not cause a "high." It is, however, abused in some situations. An emerging pattern of abuse is a combination of heroin and cocaine. Cocaine gives a rapid but short term high, whereas heroin is long lasting. This is a particularly intractable problem (Grinspoon & Bakala, 1988).

Etiology and Incidence

In almost all cases, dependence on these substances is a reflection of other problems in an individual's life. These may be related to a pre-existing or coexisting character disorder, situational problems, or adjustment difficulties. For example, Vietnam veterans who were substance abusers were found to have been subjected to higher levels of stress than those who were not (Penk, Robinowitz, Roberts, Patterson, Dolan, & Atkins, 1981). Since abuse of these substances requires contact with illicit sources, establishment of a dependence requires criminal/illegal action on the part of the individual. It is common, for example, to find this sort of addiction in individuals with prior histories of delinquency or from unstable home situations. It should be noted, however, that these addictions can be found in individuals from all sorts of life circumstances (Penk, et al., 1981).

Incidence appears to be roughly 0.7% of the population, i.e., this percentage of adults in the United States have abused opioids at some point in their lives (APA, 1987).

Prognosis

Dependence on these drugs is intractable, although apparently less so than cocaine. The drugs cause significant tolerance effects fairly rapidly, and withdrawal symptoms are severe and unpleasant. Thus, after initial experiences with the drugs for the "high" they cause, later experiences are often attempts to avoid withdrawal symptoms. In addition, since these drugs are related to lifestyle and personality characteristics, the environment tends to support the addiction. To successfully withdraw, individuals may have to cope not only with withdrawal but also with making necessary changes in lifestyle to avoid social pressure to continue abusing the substance. Tolerance for the drugs is a particular problem. As it develops, increasing amounts are required to experience the euphoria it causes. However, these drugs are also CNS depressants. Many individuals die of overdoses, particularly of heroin.

Although prognosis is generally thought to be poor, there is not absolute agreement on this. Cottrell, Childs-Clarke, and Ghodse (1985) found that less than half of a group of 83 drug abusers were still using heroin/methadone 11 years later. Among those individuals, deviant behavior had diminished. As with other abuse, coexisting psychosis is a predictor of poor prognosis (Perkins, Simpson, & Tsuang, 1986).

Implications for Function and Treatment

These addictions have a particularly severe impact on function. The drugs are illicit and expensive and tolerance develops quickly. Thus, individuals who become dependent on these substances are likely to spend much of their time in pursuit of their next "fix." Once ingested, the drugs cause lethargy and withdrawal, making it difficult for the individual to maintain stable employment. The need for money to purchase the drug, accompanied by its effects, means that these individuals often turn to crime as a means to support a habit. Theft and prostitution are common among addicts.

In addition to impact on ability to maintain vocational function, dependence has a severe impact on social function. Social life also focuses on the drug, friends tend to be involved, and relationships are tenuous as the drug assumes primary importance in the individual's life. Similarly, leisure activities are replaced by the drug, which becomes the individual's vocation, avocation, and social life.

ADL and IADL function become impaired as dependence increases. The lethargy while under the influence of the drug leads to lessened interest in self-maintenance and maintenance of the surroundings. Individuals may have little interest in appearance and hygiene or in the environment. In addition, financial woes tend to be severe, leaving little for food, shelter, or clothing.

Treatment often begins in inpatient settings. "Cold turkey" withdrawal is held by some to be most effective, i.e., the individual must simply stop taking the substance, rather than withdrawing from it gradually. For most individuals, withdrawal is aided by use of medications such as methadone, which is discussed below. Medical management may be necessary to deal with complications of withdrawal. A dilemma with this sort of treatment is that some individuals use it as a way to lower their tolerance for the drug, so that when they leave the inpatient setting, their dose requirement of the drug will be less. At the same time, other interventions must be made. Approaches similar to AA have been reported to be successful with some individuals.

In some cases, outpatient treatment may be an option. Methadone, which can cause dependence if taken in an unsupervised setting, is often used as a mechanism for withdrawing individuals from opioids. It prevents the withdrawal symptoms, without providing a "high." However, once started, it must be continued, or withdrawal symptoms will occur. Methadone is generally administered in highly structured settings that require the individual to come in regularly to obtain the drug and psychotherapeutic interventions. Those who finish treatment tend to remain abstinent (Stimmel, Goldberg, Ratkopf, & Cohen, 1977).

Social circumstances also affect outcomes. Those individuals who have supportive and involved families do better than others (Kosten, Jalali, Hogan, & Kleber, 1983). This is problematic, however, as opioid addiction often involves a whole lifestyle supported and encouraged by the social system.

Implications for Occupational Therapy

Approaches to individuals with opioid addictions are similar to those used with alcoholics. Intervention focuses on substitution of acceptable activities for those involved with obtaining and using the drug. In addition, expression of feelings, building of self-confidence and self-esteem, and stress reduction are important, and may all be accompanied through activity.

As with other types of substance abuse, vocational performance is often impaired. These individuals may need to learn or relearn work-related behaviors through occupational therapy interventions.

Cannabis

This is probably the most commonly used illicit substance, and it is popularly conceived as one of the less dangerous drugs. Many individuals begin using marijuana and hashish in social settings, believing them to be relatively harmless. Psychoactive symptoms appear to be less than those of other substances, making it unlikely that individuals with dependence will be seen in treatment. Chronic cannabis use seems to interfere with motivation and therefore with function. In addition, a fairly high proportion of individuals with other psychiatric disturbances and alcoholics are also problematic cannabis abusers and these individuals have a much worse course.

Dependence and abuse generally develop over a relatively long period. They are characterized by increasing frequency of use, rather than increased amounts at a given time. Prolonged use may lead to lethargy, anhedonia, and memory and attention deficits. Some changes in perceptual skills have also been noted. However, function is not as severely impaired as in other forms of substance abuse.

Data about marijuana use are conflicting. Although some researchers have found most mental processes to be impaired in experienced cannabis users (Klonoff, Low, & Marcus, 1973), others have noted such changes only in those who are not experienced users (Weil, Zinberg, & Nelsen, 1968). Weil and colleagues (1968) found impairment only on digit symbol and pursuit rotor performance in their naive subjects; experienced subjects had no performance decrements.

Kandel (1984) found that marijuana users were more likely to abuse other substances and to have poorer adjustment to normal adult roles. They were more likely to participate in deviant activities and to have psychiatric hospitalizations. It is unclear, however, whether the marijuana led to deviant behavior or the reverse.

There is one situation in which cannabis poses clear risk, and that is in schizophrenics (Treffert, 1978). Schizophrenic users are very likely to have psychotic episodes requiring hospitalization as a result of this use. In addition, it has been noted that cannabis is the second step in a heirarchy of abuse for adolescents (Kandel & Faust, 1975). Although not all adolescents who use cannabis will go on to other drugs, such new abuse is more likely among those who do.

Inhalants

A wide variety of substances may be inhaled, including gasoline, paint thinners, glue, and various cleaners. The active ingredients are aliphatic and aromatic hydrocarbons that cause intoxication, resulting in a "high." This type of substance abuse most often appears in children and adolescents, particularly those from disadvantaged backgrounds. These children are typically from dysfunctional families and show significant adjustment problems including truancy, poor grades, and delinquency. It appears that their adjustment problems predate the substance abuse. It also appears that abuse of inhalants leads to abuse of other substances. Inhalants are extremely dangerous, leading to physical and mental problems, including kidney and liver disease, even when used for only short periods.

Tolerance and withdrawal symptoms have been reported, but it is not clear that either phenomenon occurs. It is clear, however, that this type of abuse is intractable, recurring even after treatment. Furthermore, the effects of the drugs exacerbate existing functional difficulties. Performance of vocational, leisure, and self-care are all affected, probably with some coexisting decrements in cognitive and psychological skills due to CNS damage.

Nicotine

Nicotine is the drug that makes cigarette smoking appealing. It is a highly addicting substance. It is a mild stimulant that is difficult to stop once an addiction has developed, usually over the course of time.

While some individuals are able to withdraw from smoking, the majority have considerable difficulty doing so. Behavioral techniques have been found to be effective in highly motivated individuals, but for many the effects of nicotine are too reinforcing to be given up.

For most, however, symptoms and interference with function are minimal, at least from a psychological perspective. Some individuals may begin to have problems in work situations as smoking is increasingly prohibited. Most, however, continue to perform well. Major problems with this type of addiction are physical, and appear over long periods. Development of lung, larynx, and oral cancer, as well as cardiovascular problems, is common, but usually occurs after decades of smoking. Such long term hazards tend to be disregarded by smokers or to provide insufficient motivation to stop a severe addiction. Other hazards, e.g., fire from careless smoking, are less well publicized. It does appear that some CNS function is compromised, possibly leading to such problems as auto accidents.

Implications for Occupational Therapy

As can be seen, substance abuse interferes with accomplishment of ADL/IADL, vocational, and leisure activities. In addition, there is reason to believe that CNS processing is impaired by some of the substances discussed above. Thus, intervention must occur at the level of both skill and performance.

Van Deusen (1989) discusses the impact of alcohol abuse on fine motor skills, tactile and figure-ground perception, and visual-spatial function. She notes that there seems to be some spontaneous recovery of these skills in individuals who abstain from drinking but that practice may enhance this recovery. Thus, her recommendation is that occupational therapy focus on remediating motor and sensory-motor deficits by way of sports activities, computer games, and so on. It is reasonable to assume that other substance abusers might respond to similar intervention.

A second area of focus for intervention is expression of emotion. Many substance abusers have difficulty verbalizing their feelings, and the expressive arts (e.g., drawing, painting) have been suggested as a modality (Smith & Glickstein, 1980). Individuals who use drugs to block emotion may benefit.

A third area of concern is use of time, in particular, leisure time (Van Deusen, 1989). Substance abuse often becomes the primary focus of activity, and these individuals need to learn through education and experimentation about alternative uses of time. The issue of time use is closely related to sociocultural considerations about work and work skills. Many substance abusers lose their jobs because of their addiction and must relearn job skills as well as work-related skills such as following directions and relating to supervisors.

More problematic is the issue of individuals who turn to substance abuse specifically because they feel hopeless about future prospects. In inner city areas, substance abusers often have no job experience or skills and no hope of acquiring them. Training in work and work-related skills may mean starting at square one with reading and writing. Although this approach can be very valuable, it is time and cost intensive. Linkage with community services and constant follow up is vital.

All these difficulties contribute to, or are caused by, poor self-esteem. Experiences that can provide both motivation and hope are essential.

Figure 5-2
Psychoactive Substance Abuse Disorders

Disorder	Symptoms	Functional Deficits
Dependence	1. Increasing use of substance	Vocational Social Leisure
	2. Focus on obtaining substance	Possibly ADL/IADL Possibly cognitive, motor, sensory motor, sensory, psychological
	3. Tolerance	May be mild to severe

Figure 5-2 *continued*
Psychoactive Substance Abuse Disorders

Disorder	Symptoms	Functional Deficits
Abuse	1. Continued substance use despite knowledge that problems are occurring 2. At least 1 month duration	As above, usually less global and less persistent

References

Allgulander, C., Borg, S., Vikander, B. (1984). A 4-6 year follow-up of 50 patients with primary dependence on sedative and hypnotic drugs. *American Journal of Psychiatry, 141,* 1580-1582.

American Psychiatric Association. (1987). *Diagnostic and Statistical Manual* 3rd ed., rev. Washington, DC: author.

Berglund, M. (1984). Suicide in alcoholism. *Archives of General Psychiatry, 41,* 888-891.

Cohen, M.J., Schandler, S.L., & Naliboff, B.D. (1983). Psychophysiological measures from intoxicated and detoxified alcoholics. *Journal of Studies on Alcohol, 44,* 271-282.

Cottrell, D., Childs-Clarke, A., & Ghodse, A.H. (1985). British opiate addicts: An 11-year follow-up. *British Journal of Psychiatry, 146,* 448-450.

Goodwin, D.W. (1985). Alcoholism and genetics: The sins of the fathers. *Archives of General Psychiatry, 42,* 171-174.

Gottheil, E., Thornton, C.C., Skoloda, T.E., & Alterman, A.I. (1982). Follow-up of abstinent and nonabstinent alcoholics. *American Journal of Psychiatry, 139,* 560-565.

Govriti, G.A. (1989). Now to fight the drug war. *The Atlantic Monthly, 263*(1), 70-76.

Grinspoon, L. & Bakalar, J. (1988). Substance use disorders. In A.M. Napoli (Ed.), *The Harvard Guide to Psychiatry.* Cambridge, MA: Belknap Press, pp. 418-433.

Kandel, D.B. (1984). Marijuana users in young adulthood. *Archives of General Psychiatry, 41,* 200-209.

Kandel, D. & Faust, R. (1975). Sequence and stages in patterns of adolescent drug use. *Archives of General Psychiatry, 32,* 923-932.

Klonoff, H., Low, M., & Marcus, A. (1973). Neuropsychological effects of marijuana. *Canadian Medical Association Journal, 108,* 150-156, 165.

Kosten, T.R., Jalali, B., Hogan, I., & Kleber, H.D. (1983). Family denial as a prognostic factor in opiate addict treatment outcome. *Journal of Nervous and Mental Disease, 171,* 611-616.

Naditch, M.P. & Fenwick, S. (1977). LSD flashbacks and ego functioning. *Journal of Abnormal Psychology, 86,* 352-359.

Penk, W.E., Robinowitz, Roberts, W.R., Patterson, E.T., Dolan, M.P., & Atkins, H.S. (1981). Adjustment differences among male substance abusers varying in degree of combat experience in Vietnam. *Journal of Consulting and Clinical Psychology, 49,* 426-437.

Perkins, K.A., Simpson, J.C., & Tsuang, M.T. (1986). Ten-year follow-up of drug abusers with acute or chronic psychosis. *Hospital and Community Psychiatry, 37,* 581-484.

Polich, J.M., Armor, D.J., & Braiker, H.B. (1980). *The Course of Alcoholism: Four Years After Treatment.* Santa Monica, CA: Rand Corporation.

Smith, T.M. & Glickstein, C.S. (1980). Art as a therapeutic modality for individuals with alcohol related problems in a milieu setting. *Occupational Therapy in Mental Health, 1*(4), 33-44.

Stimmel, B., Goldberg, J., Rotkopf, E., & Cohen, M. (1977). Ability to remain abstinent after methadone detoxification. *Journal of American Medical Association, 237,* 1216-1220.

Treffert, D.A. (1978). Marijuana use in schizophrenia: A clear hazard. *American Journal of Psychiatry, 135,* 1213-1215.

Vaillant, G.E. (1988). The alcohol-dependent and drug-dependent person. In A.M. Nicholi (Ed.), *The New Harvard Guide to Psychiatry.* Cambridge, MA: Belknap Press, pp. 700-713.

Van Deusen, J. (1989). Alcohol abuse and perceptual-motor dysfunction: The occupational therapist's role. *American Journal of Occupational Therapy, 43,* 384-390.

Washton, A.M., Gold, M.S., Pattash, A.C., & Semlitz, L. (1984). Adolescent cocaine abusers. *The Lancet, September 29,* 746.

Weil, A.T., Zinberg, N.E., & Nelson, J.M. (1968). Clinical and psycholgoical effects of marijuana in man. *Science, 162,* 1234-1242.

Yamaguchi, K. & Kandel, D.B. (1984). Patterns of drug use from adolescence to young adulthood: III. Predictors of progression. *American Journal of Public Health, 74,* 673-680.

Chapter 6
Schizophrenia, Paranoid Disorders and Other Psychoses

The psychotic disorders, including schizophrenia, are among the most disabling psychiatric conditions, and perhaps for that reason have received a great deal of attention. The clinical definition of schizophrenia has been narrowed considerably in the most recent diagnostic manuals, resulting, among other things, in a poorer prognosis for the disorders (Harrow, Carone, & Westermeyer, 1985). Because people diagnosed as schizophrenic now are more likely to really have the constellation of schizophrenic symptoms, they are those who are likely to have poor outcomes. *DSM-III-R* has identified several characteristics that must be present for the diagnosis to be made, reflecting a minimum duration and a specific constellation of symptoms.

Figure 6-1
Common Types of Schizophrenia

* Catatonic
* Disorganized
* Undifferentiated
* Residual
* Paranoid

Schizophrenia

This is one of the disorders defined relative to function. For the diagnosis to be made, functional level must be below the highest level previously achieved. In addition, thought, including both content and form, is disturbed. Content refers to what a thought is about, e.g., snakes, evil spirits, red balloons. Form refers to the way in which thoughts are put together. Someone who is schizophrenic might see red balloons turning into fire, then suddenly begin to see demons emerging from walls. Delusions, beliefs that are firmly held but not true, are frequently found in these individuals. The most common types of delusions are delusions of persecution (fear that one is being followed or will be harmed by others), delusions of reference (the belief that one is being talked about by others), or delusions of grandeur (the belief that one possesses special powers, abilities, or gifts). Loosening of associations, incoherence, or excessively concrete or abstract thought are also characteristic. Someone with these symptoms might answer a question about the weather by launching into a discussion of weather patterns in outer space or by making an unintelligible response. An excessively concrete response might be that there are two rain drops on the window of a red car outside, an excessively abstract answer might be that weather is in the eye of the beholder and relates to the meaning of life.

Perception and affect are also disturbed. Hallucinations, experiences such as hearing voices or feeling ants crawling under the skin, are typical. Auditory hallucinations (hearing voices) are most common, although any sense may be involved. For example, the individual may smell peculiar smells and think that poison gas is in the room or see strange figures in the mirror. Affect is either flat or inappropriate. Some of these individuals are totally expressionless, whereas others may have bizarre smiles, laugh inappropriately, and so on.

Peculiar psychomotor behavior may be present. Odd mannerisms, grimacing, hyperactivity or, conversely, waxy rigidity may be observed. Sense of self is also impaired. The individual may have difficulty discriminating between self and others or between self and the environment.

Most often, the disorder appears during adolescence or early adulthood. Masterson (1967) found that symptomatic adolescents followed for 5 years did not "grow out" of their problems. Less often, the schizophrenia develops later in life. For the diagnosis to be made, symptoms must exist for at least 6 months, and typically the disorder continues for years. It is usually characterized by a prodromal phase, in which function begins to deteriorate. The individual withdraws from friends and family, and work, self-care, and avocational activities suffer. The individual may begin to have trouble relating to people at work or school, to stop bathing, and to spend most free time staring in a mirror or just sitting. One individual with schizophrenia reported spending most of her time watching TV to receive "important messages from powers above." The active phase is characterized by delusions and hallucinations, thought disorder, and other psychotic symptoms. This phase may occur spontaneously or as a result of stress. The residual phase is the third phase. It is often similar to the prodromal phase in terms of symptomatology. During this phase functional level continues to be below the highest level ever achieved by the individual. Most individuals continue to have flat affect, peculiar behavior, and functional difficulties between active phases. They usually have few friends or interests, ignore self-care, and may have problems concentrating well enough to work.

Several types of schizophrenia are identified in *DSM-III-R*, with slightly differing constellations of symptoms. Catatonic schizophrenia is characterized by stupor, rigidity, peculiar posturing, or catatonic excitement, i.e., motor excitation that is purposeless and not affected by external stimuli. Individuals with catatonic schizophrenia may sit rigid for hours without moving, often in positions that appear very uncomfortable. They may not eat, speak, or in any way acknowledge the environment during these periods.

Disorganized type is characterized by incoherence, flat or inappropriate affect, and disorganization of behavior. Undifferentiated schizophrenia or residual schizophrenia may be the label applied when catatonic or disorganized categories do not fit the individual. Individuals who are diagnosed undifferentiated schizophrenia are usually unkempt and disheveled, walk with a shuffling gait and stooped posture, and may mutter unintelligibly. Conversations with such individuals may be incomprehensible or they may exclaim with great fear about voices telling them terrible things or frightening figures appearing to them. They tend to be lethargic and difficult to engage in activity, or occasionally to be excessively active but not engaged in any purposeful activity.

Paranoid type is noticeably different from the other schizophrenias, as catatonic behavior, inappropriate affect, disorganized behavior, and loose associations are not present. The presenting feature is a well-developed delusional system in which persecutory delusions feature prominently. If hallucinations are present, they are usually auditory and often feed into the sense of persecution these individuals experience. These are the individuals who, if willing to discuss their fears at all, may complain of being followed by the FBI, for example. One woman called the police daily to complain that her neighbors were pumping poison gas into her hourse. Another felt that people wanted to kill him because he "knew the secret of world peace."

Etiology and Incidence

There are a variety of theories about the emergence of schizophrenia. There is a family pattern that can be demonstrated even when the individual is not raised by the biological family. Thus a genetic component is evident (Guze, Cloninger, Martin, & Clayton, 1983). Individuals with close relatives with schizophrenia have a 3.2% risk (Tsuang, Winokur, & Crowe, 1980) as compared with a risk of less than 0.6% for the general population. Monozygotic (identical) twins have up to six times the normal risk (Gottesman & Shields, 1972).

However, the genetic component does not seem sufficient to cause the emergence of the disease, since not all individuals who are genetically predisposed develop schizophrenia, even if they are identical twins. Some theorists suggest that environmental factors including a variety of psychosocial stressors, such as maladjusted family relationships, contribute as well. Stress has been examined as an etiologic factor, and although it seems unlikely that it causes schizophrenia, it appears to be a factor in exacerbations (Tsuang, Faraone, and Day, 1988). Dohrenwend and Egri (1981) feel it is a significant contributing factor in the emergence of the disease. There is evidence that the diagnosis is more common in lower socioeconomic groups, but this may occur as an outcome of the disease rather than as a predisposing factor. Since the disease is marked by functional decline, the individual may move downward in terms of socioeconomic factors. It appears that premorbid social anhedonia (Mishlove & Chapman, 1985) and poor interpersonal competence (Beckfield, 1985) are associated with schizophrenia.

Recent explanations have focused on biological factors in schizophrenia. A variety of studies have examined the role of biochemical changes, neurological factors, and other physical agents in the emergence of the disorder. Conflicting findings in this sphere have led some to theorize that schizophrenia may be more than one disease (Kety & Matthysse, 1988). Biological factors discussed include brain abnormalities, genetic disorders and neurotransmitter disorders (Tsuang et al, 1980) as well as the possibility of an autoimmune disorder (Knight, 1985).

Another biological factor examined in some detail is the role of neurotransmitters. The phenothiazines, drugs commonly used to treat psychotic disorders, block dopamine receptors (Carlson & Lindqvist, 1974), suggesting elevated dopamine transmission as a causative factor. In addition, structural abnormalities have been found in the brains of some schizophrenic individuals. Ventricular enlargement has been noted (Andreasen, Smith, Jacoby, Denners, & Olsen, 1982), although the frequency and impact of this finding have been debated. In addition, individuals with schizophrenia tend to have smaller frontal lobes, cerebrums, and crania, suggesting early developmental abnormalities (Andreasen, Nasrallah, Dunn, Olson, Brove, Ehrhardt, et al, 1986).

Prevalence of schizophrenia is approximately 1% of the adult population (APA, 1987). Full-blown catatonic schizophrenia is the least common, but its symptoms may be seen in other forms of schizophrenia (Abrams & Taylor, 1976). Women are affected more often than men (Tsuang, Tohen, and Murphy, 1988).

Prognosis

In most instances, it is probable that function will be impaired over long periods. Thus, for many individuals, the prognosis for schizophrenia must be considered poor. Tsuang, Woolson, Winokur, and Crowe (1981) found schizophrenia to be a stable diagnosis over 30 to 40 years. While the diagnosis is stable, it seems that as individuals age some of the symptoms are ameliorated. Some diminution of function continues, but this may become less prominent over time. The individual may have fewer active episodes, and remain in the residual phase for long periods.

A distinction relative to prognosis has also been made with regard to premorbid personality and onset of the disorder. In some individuals, premorbid function was good, and emergence of the disorder can be clearly linked with a specific set of psychosocial stressors. One woman, for example, held a secretarial job, had a husband, and rather suddenly began to hallucinate. This occurred shortly after she was laid off from work. Such individuals appear to have relatively good prognoses. They may have one or several episodes of active symptoms, and then return to premorbid levels of function. When onset is more insidious, and less obviously linked to stress, and when premorbid function was less than optimal, the course of the disease is more malignant, with poorer probable outcome (Bleuler, 1978). A young adolescent who does poorly in school, has few friends, and is labeled by others as "strange" may later develop schizophrenia. In this case, prognosis is poor.

A number of researchers have discussed factors that seem to predict outcome. Stephens, Astrup, and Mangrum (1966) found that good prognosis correlated with acute onset, presence of a clear precipitating factor, no family history, normal IQ, and good premorbid adjustment. Roff (1974) added absence of a disturbed family member to this list. Kendler and Tsuang (1988) note that a family history of unipolar illness is more common in "good prognosis" schizophrenics.

It appears that roughly 25% of schizophrenics recover (Bleuler, 1978; Cutting, 1986) while somewhere between 10% and 25% become severe and chronic. It is worth mentioning that some believe that if the client recovers he or she was not truly schizophrenic (Leonhard, 1966).

Implications for Function and Treatment

As noted, functional impairment is a defining characteristic of schizophrenia. Social, vocational, avocational, and self-care abilities are markedly affected, leading to a global picture of disability. It is important to note, however, that the degree of impairment is variable, dependent on severity of the illness, phase, and type of schizophrenia.

During the prodromal and residual phases, functional ability may be minimally impaired. This is particularly true where supportive treatment such as outpatient counseling is available. Individuals who can identify environments in which demand and stress are reduced may do well. Such individuals may regain reasonable measures of social and self-care function. In addition, if a supportive work environment can be found, one with low levels of stress and an understanding supervisor, they may be able to hold jobs.

For other individuals, however, the prodromal and residual phases are characterized more by functional impairment than by psychological symptoms. Thus, even though their delusions and hallucinations may disappear and their thought processes clear, they may continue to demonstrate severe social and vocational impairment. This is particularly true for individuals whose premorbid functioning was poor. As noted in an earlier section, individuals who develop schizophrenia often were isolated, anhedonic (lacking the ability to enjoy events), and lacking in motivation prior to the onset of the disorder. An additional factor in probable level of function during the residual phase is the time of onset of the disorder. If the individual develops schizophrenia during adolescence, he or she may miss important milestones in normal development. This makes it more difficult to function well later, even when acute symptoms abate.

As an example, a young adult who was isolated and lethargic as a teenager, had few friends, and did poorly in school might develop schizophrenia and, even during the residual phase, continue to have few friends and find work difficult. By contrast, someone who held a job, had a social circle, and developed schizophrenia in his or her late 20s would be likely to do much better during residual phases.

During active phases of the disease, functional impairment is much more severe. It is rare that these individuals can work, they demonstrate very little motivation to engage in other activities, and they tend to be severely withdrawn socially. Personal hygiene suffers, as do other self-care activities.

Impairments among individuals with schizophrenia occur at the skill level, as well as the performance level, probably contributing to the overall poor function noted. A whole variety of cognitive decrements have been found. IQ is thought to be lower among schizophrenics (Aylward, Walker, & Bettes, 1984; Schwartzman, Douglass & Muir, 1962) and to become worse as the disease progresses. This is most prominent in hospitalized individuals but is true of others as well.

Among the other cognitive impairments noted are disturbances of will and volition (Frith, 1987), poor spatial and nonspatial associative learning (Kemali, Maj, Galderisi, Monteleone, & Mucci, 1987), difficulty with color perception (David, 1987), and poverty of written response (Manschreck, Ames, Maher, & Schneyer, 1987).

Taylor and Abrams (1984) found moderate to severe global cognitive impairment, which they later divided into two subtypes (Taylor & Abrams, 1987). One pattern is a bifrontal and nondominant hemisphere dysfunction, impacting personality and affect among other factors, the other, dominant temporo-parietal-occipital, impacting on the senses and ability to process sensory information. This second pattern is consistent with symptoms of thought disorder.

Other dysfunctions identified include poor visuomotor tracking (Gaebel &

Ulrich, 1987) even during periods of remission, and disturbed voluntary motor performance (Manschreck, Maher, Rucklos, & Vereen, 1982).

Unfortunately, all these problems are compounded when tardive dyskinesia appears as a side effect of psychopharmacologic treatment (DeWolfe, Ryan, & Wolf, 1988). Motor performance, sensory processing, learning, and reasoning are all even worse in these individuals, and IQ appears to be affected as well. In addition, long term hospitalization may also have a negative impact on these skills, particularly IQ.

An additional skill area of particular importance is the social sphere. As noted earlier, poor social skills may be among the predictors of schizophrenia. This is a good prognostic indicator, as well (Morrison & Bellack, 1987). During periods of florid illness, social skills may be almost totally absent, and even during remission social interactions may be awkward, unskilled, or contentious.

An exception to this picture is noted among individuals with paranoid schizophrenia. These individuals tend to be much better organized and to demonstrate less cognitive impairment even during active phases of the disease. They may be able to work, are usually reasonably competent in self-care activities, and may even have avocational interests (although those activities might relate to escaping persecution, building "security systems" for the home, for example). Social functioning is impaired as a result of persecutory fears, but superficial social skills are often maintained. Work and social activities are interfered with as a result of suspicions, which often lead to angry exchanges with supervisors and neighbors who are believed to harbor wishes to harm the individual. These fears may be well masked, however. In some cases, the masking is symptomatic of the disorder, as the individual does not trust anyone enough to confide about his or her concerns.

Schizophrenia is generally treated through a combination of modalities. It is a disorder in which psychotropic drugs are clearly effective (Tsuang et al, 1988). These drugs are useful in minimizing thought disorder and sensory impairment during the active phase of the illness. In addition, medication may be administered over long periods to reduce the probability of exacerbations and to lengthen the intervals between active periods of the disease. Issues related to use of medication for these disorders is discussed further in Chapter 11.

Other treatments include behavior, environmental, and social interventions. During the active period of the disorder, individuals with schizophrenia often require hospitalization. While drug treatment is instituted, the individual may also be placed in a therapeutic milieu or in some sort of behavioral program. Brief hospital stays seem beneficial, particularly if community follow up is available (Caffey, Galbrecht, & Klett, 1971). Milieu therapy, in which the whole environment has been structured to provide specific therapeutic effects, has semed to benefit nonchronic schizophrenics more than those who are chronic (Gunderson, 1980).

In addition, skill training is often introduced. Many of these individuals never had the opportunity to acquire skills because symptoms of the disorder intervened in the normal developmental process. Others, typically who have been hospitalized frequently or for long periods, lose skills as a result of environmental deprivation. Social skills training is a patterned set of interventions designed to assist individuals in enhancing relationships. It has been developed as a way to deal with the frequent social impairment noted in individuals with schizophrenia. Research on the subject suggests that social skills training can improve specific behaviors, but has less impact on overall quality of life (Wallace, Nelson, Liberman, Aitchison, Lukoff, Elder, et al, 1980).

ADL and IADL training may also be employed. Vocational assessment and work skills training are also part of intervention, particularly as individuals prepare for discharge. Work as an activity is clearly important as an intervention (Bebbington & Kuipers, 1982).

A variety of types of psychotherapy, individual and group, have been attempted with schizophrenics, with reports of varying degrees of success. Although Freud specifically noted that psychoanalysis was not useful with schizophrenics, it has nonetheless been attempted. Other forms of verbal therapy have also been employed, largely as adjuncts to more structured treatments and medication.

In addition, family therapy is often employed, both to assist the family in dealing with the problem and to remediate psychosocial stressors related to family interaction. Some theorists have suggested that schizophrenia is a rational adaptation to an irrational environment (cf, Henry, 1956 and Laing, 1969). The correlate to this belief is the need to treat the environment as well as the individual. It seems clear that family interactions are important in development of the disorder (Doane, Falloon, Goldstein, & Mintz, 1985). Thus, family therapy is a logical choice for intervention. Studies have found it to be helpful, particularly in combination with other approaches (Hogarty, Anderson, Reiss, Kornblith, Greenwald, Javna, et al, 1986; Falloon, Boyd, McGill, Williamson, Razani, Moss, et al, 1985).

During the prodromal and residual phases of the disease, a variety of approaches are employed to minimize risk of exacerbation. Medications may be continued, though it is not uncommon for the individual to stop taking the drug. In some instances, this appears to be sufficient to cause the disease to enter its active phase.

A variety of environmental supports have been developed. Among the environmental supports are community mental health centers that provide ongoing therapy, medication, and social support. Some schizophrenics do well in sheltered environments such as group homes and sheltered workshops. Halfway houses may ease the transition to the community.

Issues relative to managment of individuals with schizophrenia in the community have received increasing notice in recent years. In the early 1960s, a move began toward deinstitutionalization of individuals with schizophrenia and other chronically mental illnesses. The original intent of this move was quite humane and logical. Prior to that time, long term institutionalization, often lasting throughout the individual's life, was common. The idea for the change related to a desire to maximize function and quality of life for these patients. The development of community mental health centers, which occurred at the same time, was intended as a means for providing support for these individuals as they returned to their communities.

The realities of deinstitutionalization have proved less satisfactory, however (Basuk & Gerson, 1978). Funding for community programs has been cut, and other bridges to the community have been slow to develop. Communities have been less than welcoming of these initiatives as the patients may continue to demonstrate peculiar behaviors. In addition, fears that individuals with schizophrenia may be dangerous are common among the general population. Although these fears do not appear to be borne out by reality, they have led to resistance to establishment of group homes and halfway houses. In some situations where extensive community education and support programs have been implemented, outcomes are more positive (Denner, 1974; Braum, Kochansky, Shapiro, Greenberg, Gudeman, Johnson, et al, 1981).

Thus, after being discharged from inpatient care, individuals with schizophrenia or other chronic mental illnesses often end up in boarding houses, nursing homes, or in the streets. These individuals may express preference for institutionalization (Drake & Wallach, 1979). The growing problem of the homeless is, at least in part, a problem caused by deinstitutionalization. Not only have community supports remained scarce, funds for inpatient treatment have been cut. Length of stay in inpatient settings has been drastically reduced, meaning that some of these individuals may be discharged prematurely. For many, a "revolving door" pattern of admissions is apparent. They are admitted, treated, and discharged, are unable to cope in the community, and must be readmitted.

It is important to note that the problems of deinstitutionalization relate to any of the chronic mental disorders, not just to schizophrenia. Individuals with chronic depression, with manic depressive disorders, and substance abuse disorders, among others, may have chronic courses that present intervention difficulties similar to those described above.

Implications for Occupational Therapy

Like many of the organic mental disorders, schizophrenia affects all performance areas and most underlying skills. Because of this, occupational therapy intervention must be comprehensive. Careful assessment must be made of motor, sensory and sensorimotor, and psychosocial skills. History of performance in self-care, leisure, and work, as well as current status should also be assessed.

As with other disorders, it is important for the occupational therapist to determine strengths as well as weaknesses. There is a tendency to ignore strengths when dealing with someone who has a disorder with a poor prognosis, but often important assets do exist that can be built upon in treatment. For example, one patient who was schizophrenic was quite artistic and creative. As he improved, he was able to find work as a greeting card artist for a company noted for its somewhat "off the wall" cards.

Another young woman with a long history of psychosis simply decided one day that the other patients on her ward at the state hospital were depressing, and that she did not want to be like them. Her recovery was long and arduous, but she eventually went back to school and became a highly effective psychotherapist. Her case illustrates, among other things, the importance of motivation as a crucial asset.

Motivating clients is no easy matter, as many are quite discouraged. Frequently, careful probing is necessary to uncover the activity that continues to have meaning for the person and the ways in which that activity can be therapeutic. For the woman described above, school was that activity. She wanted to understand as much as possible about her own condition.

Remediating skill deficits through education, behavioral approaches, sensorimotor approaches, etc., is vital. The client discussed above was almost totally incapable of social interaction. She had to learn to make eye contact, engage in social interaction, and so on before she could consider going to school.

Not only must skills and performance be remediated, but self-esteem must be addressed. As noted, these individuals often feel a profound sense of despair. Activities that provide success and social reinforcement (making simple cookies for others on the unit, for example) can be quite helpful.

Another dominant emotion is fear. Many hallucinations and delusions are quite frightening, as are the reactions of people in the community to these individuals, whose appearance and behavior may seem quite odd.

Transition to and maintenance in the community require considerable skill training and support for the individual. For some more severe and chronic individuals, sheltered living may be of value. At other times, relatively simple strategies are effective. A dentist who was diagnosed as paranoid schizo-phrenic was able to return to independent work and living once he learned by way of a behavioral program to discuss his delusions only with his therapist and family.

The occupational therapist should also place particular emphasis on use of leisure time. Unstructured time may be hardest for these individuals to manage.

Intervention with individuals who have schizophrenia is currently a subject of considerable debate in occupational therapists. A variety of theories have been advanced (Allen, 1985; Kielhofner, 1985; King, 1974). It is beyond the scope of this text to deal with this debate, but therapists should familiarize themselves with the various theories and the evidence that supports or refutes each.

Delusional Disorder

As with paranoid schizophrenia, the primary feature of this disorder is the existence of a persistent, nonbizarre delusion. The diagnosis is made only in the absence of any identifiable organic problem that caused the disorder. The delusion may have any content, most prominent being erotomanic, in which the individual believes that he or she is loved by someone else, usually a prominent figure whom the individual does not actually know; grandiose, a belief that the individual has some special, great characteristic; jealous, in which the individual is convinced that a spouse or lover is unfaithful; persecutory, a belief that the individual is being conspired against; or somatic, a belief that the individual has some gross physical problem. Persecutory delusions are most common.

The disorder most often occurs in middle or later life and is more common among deaf or immigrant individuals. Cause is not established, although it appears that the deaf or those who do not speak English as a first language may misconstrue what is said by others and make negative interpretations of motives.

The course of the disease is variable, although most commonly chronic, with exacerbations and remissions. Impairment of vocational, avocational, and self-care performance is rare, whereas social impairment is frequent and often severe.

Other Psychotic Disorders

There are several categories of diagnosis that are made when the disorder does not fit the criteria for schizophrenia, paranoid disorder, or mood disorders that have psychotic features. In particular, these diagnoses may be made when criteria of duration, symptom constellation, or functional impairment are not met. They include brief reactive psychosis, a label applied when the psychosis clearly relates to a psychosocial stressor and is of brief (1 month maximum) duration. Schizophreniform disorder is identical to schizophrenia, without meeting the criterion of duration. Thus, any psychosis that manifests with schizophrenia-like symptoms, but lasts from 1 to 6 months, will be called schizophreniform. If this persists for 6 months, the diagnosis will be changed to schizophrenia.

Schizoaffective disorder does not meet the criteria for either schizophrenia or a psychotic mood disorder, but has characteristics of both. In many ways it represents a midpoint between these disorders. For example, the course of the disease is typically chronic, but prognosis is better than for schizophrenia, worse than for a mood disorder.

Finally, induced psychotic disorder is the label employed when a psychosis occurs as a result of association with someone else who is psychotic. Most typically an individual will be drawn into the delusional system of a significant other. In these cases, impairment is not as severe as for the first individual, but the disorder is amenable to treatment only if the relationship can be altered.

None of these disorders is well understood and etiological factors are not clear. Although all have better prognoses than schizophrenia, the course of each is variable. Treatment is employed on the basis of symptoms exhibited, with drugs, hospitalization, psychotherapy, behavioral therapy, and so on being attempted with varying degrees of success.

Figure 6-2
Schizophrenia

Disorder	Symptoms	Functional Deficits
Schizophrenia	1. Delusions 2. Catatonia 3. Hallucinations 4. Flat or inappropriate affect 5. Episodic deterioration of function 6. Continuous symptoms of varing severity over at least 6 months	Global, with exacerbations
A. Catatonic type	1. Catatonia is most marked symptom	Global, with exacerbations
B. Disorganized	1. Previous symptoms plus incoherence or severely disorganized behavior	Global, with exacerbations

Figure 6-2 *continued*
Schizophrenia

Disorder	Symptoms	Functional Deficits
C. Paranoid	1. Well formed delusional system 2. Absence of loose associations, flat or inappropriate affect, catatonic or disorganized behavior	Usually less impaired ADL/IADL Usually little motor impairment

References

Abrams, R. & Taylor, M.A. (1976). Catatonia: A prospective clinical study. *Archives of General Psychiatry, 33,* 579-581.

Allen, C. (1985). *Occupational Therapy for Psychiatric Diseases: Measurement and Management of Cognitive Diseases.* Boston: Little Brown & Co.

Andreasen, N.C., Smith, M.R., Jacoby, C.G., Dennert, J.W., & Olsen, S.A. (1982). Ventricular enlargement in schizophrenia: Definition and prevalence. *American Journal of Psychiatry, 193,* 292-296.

Andreasen, N.C., Nasrallah, H.A., Dunn, V., Olson, S.C., Brove, W.M., Ehrhardt, J.C., et al. (1986). Structural abnormalities in the frontal system in schizophrenia. *Archives of General Psychiatry, 43,* 136-144.

Aylward, E., Walker, E., & Bettes, B. (1984). Intelligence in schizophrenia: Meta-analysis of the research. *Schizophrenia Bulletin, 10,* 430-459.

Bassuk, E.L. & Gerson, S. (1978). Deinstitutionalization and mental health services. *Scientific American, 238*(2),46-53.

Bebbington, P. & Kuipers, L. (1982). Social managment of schizophrenia. *British Journal of Hospital Medicine, 28,* 399-402.

Beckfield, D.F. (1985). Interpersonal competence among college men hypothesized to be at risk for schizophrenia. *Journal of Abnormal Psychology, 94,* 397-404.

Bleuler, M.E. (1978). The long-term course of schizophrenic psychoses. In Wynne, Cromwell, & Matthysse (Eds.) *The Nature of Schizophrenia: New Approach to Research and Treatment,* pp. 631-636.

Braun, P., Kochansky, G., Shapiro, R., Greenberg, S., Gudeman, J.E., Johnson, S., et al. (1981). Overview: Deinstitutionalization of psychiatric patients, a critical review of outcome studies. *American Journal of Psychiatry, 138,* 736-749.

Caffey, E.M., Galbrecht, C.R., & Klett, C.J. (1971). Brief hospitalization and aftercare in the treatment of schizophrenia. *Archives of General Psychiatry, 24,* 81-86.

Carlson, A. & Lindqvist, M. (1974). Effect of chlorpromazine or haldioperol on formation of 3-methoxytryamine and normethanephrine in mouse brain. *Acta Pharmacologica, 20,* 140-144.

Cutting, J. (1986). Outcome in schizophrenia: Overview. In T.A. Kerr & R.P. Snaith (Eds.), *Contemporary Issues in Schizophrenia.* Washington, D.C.: American Psychiatric Press; pp. 433-440.

David, A.S. (1987). Tachistoscopic tests of colour naming and matching in schizophrenia: Evidence for posterior callosum dysfunction? *Psychological Medicine, 17,* 621-630.

Denver, B. (1974). Returning madness to an accepting community. *Community Mental Health Journal, 10,* 163-172.

DeWolfe, A.S., Ryan, J.J., & Wolf, M.W. (1988). Cognitive sequelae of tardive dyskinesia. *Journal of Nervous and Mental Disease, 176,* 270-274.

Doane, J.A., Faloon, I.R.H., Goldstein, M.J., & Mintz, J. (1985). Parental affective style and the treatment of schizophrenia. *Archives of General Psychiatry, 42,* 34-42.

Dohrenwend, B.P. & Egri, G. (1981). Recent stressful life events and episodes of schizophrenia. *Schizophrenia Bulletin, 7,* 12-23.

Drake, R.E. & Wallach, M.A. (1979). Will mental patients stay in the community? A social psychological perspective. *Journal of Consulting and Clinical Psychology, 47,* 285-294.

Falloon, I.R.H., Boyd, J.L., McGill, C., Williamson, M., Razani, J., Moss, H.B., et al. (1985). Family management in the prevention of morbidity of schizophrenia. *Archives of General Psychiatry, 42,* 887-896.

Frith, C.D. (1987). The positive and negative symptoms of schizophrenia reflect impairments in the perception and initiation of action. *Psychological Medicine, 17,* 631-648.

Gaebel, W. & Ulrich, G. (1987). Visuomotor tracking performance in schizophrenia: Relationship with psychopathological subtyping. *Neuropsychobiology, 17,* 66-71.

Gottesman, T.T. & Shields, J. (1972). *Schizophrenia and Genetics: A Twin Study Vantage Point.* New York: Academic Press.

Gunderson, J.G. (1980). A reevaluation of milieu therapy for nonchronic schizophrenic patients. *Schizophrenia Bulletin, 6,* 64-69.

Guze, S.B., Cloninger, R., Martin, R.L., & Clayton, P.J. (1983). A follow-up and family study of schizophrenia. *Archives of General Psychiatry, 40,* 1273-1276.

Harrow, M., Carone, B.J., & Westermeyer, J.F. (1985). The course of psychosis schizophrenia: Relationship with psychopathological subtyping. *Neuropsychobiology, 17,* pp. 66-71.

Henry, J. (1965). *Pathways to Madness.* New York: Vintage Press.

Hogarty, G.E., Anderson, C.M., Reiss, D.J., Kornblith, S.J., Greenwald, D.P., Javna, C.D., et al. (1986). Family psychoeducation, social skills training, and maintenance chemotherapy in the aftercare treatment of schizophrenia. *Archives of General Psychiatry, 43,* 633-642.

Kemali, D., Mario, M., Galderisi, S., Monteleone, P., & Mucci, A. (1987). Conditional associative learning in drug-free schizophrenic patients. *Neuropsychobiology, 17,* 30-34.

Kendler, K.S. & Tsuang, M.T. (1988). Outcome and familial psychopathology in schizophrenia. *Archives of General Psychiatry, 45,* 338-346.

Kety, S.S. & Matthysse, S. (1988). Genetic and biochemical aspects of schizophrenia. In Williams (Ed.) pp. 139-151.

Kielhofner, G. (Ed.) (1985). *A Model of Human Occupation: Theory and Application.* Baltimore: Williams and Wilkins.

King, L. (1974). A sensory integrative approach to schizophrenia. *American Journal of Occupational Therapy, 28,* 529-536.

Knight, J.G. (1985). Possible autoimmune mechanisms in schizophrenia, *Integrated Psychiatry, 3,* 134-143.

Laing, R.D. (1969). *The Politics of the Family.* New York: Vantage Press.

Leonhard, K. (1966). The question of prognosis in schizophrenia. *International Journal of Psychiatry, 2,* 630-635.

Manschreck, T.C., Ames, D., Maher, B.A., & Schneyer, M.L. (1987). Impoverished written responses and negative features of schizophrenia. *Perceptual and Motor Skills, 64,* 1163-1169.

Manschreck, T.C., Maher, B.A., Rucklos, M.E., & Vereen, D.R. (1982). Disturbed voluntary motor activity in schizophrenic disorder. *Psychological Medicine, 12,* 73-84.

Masterson, J.F. (1967). The symptomatic adolescent five years later: He didn't grow out of it. *American Journal of Psychiatry, 123,* 1338-1345.

Mishlove, M. & Chapman, L.J. (1985). Social anhedonia in the prediction of psychosis proneness. *Journal of Abnormal Psychology, 94,* 384-396.

Morrison, R.L. & Bellack, A.S. (1987). Social functioning of schizophrenic patients: Clinical and research issues. *Schizophrenia Bulletin, 13,* 715-725.

Roff, J.D. (1974). Adolescent schizophrenia: Variables related to differences in long-term adult outcome. *Journal of Consulting and Clinical Psychology, 42,* 180-183.

Schwartzman, A.E., Douglas, V.E., & Muir, W.R. (1962). Intellectural loss in schizophrenia: Part II. *Canadian Journal of Psychology, 16,* 161-168.

Stephens, J.H., Astrup, C., & Mangrum, J.C. (1966). Prognostic factors in recovered and deteriorated schizophrenics.

Taylor, M.A. & Abrams, R. (1984). Cognitive impairment in schizophrenia. *American Journal of Psychiatry, 141,* 196-201.

Taylor, M.A. & Abrams, R. (1987).   Cognitive impairment patterns in schizophrenia and affective disorder.   *Journal of Neurology, Neurosurgery, and Psychiatry, 50,* 895-899

Tsuang, M.T., Winokur, G., Crowe, R.R. (1980).   Morbidity risks of schizophrenia and affective disorder among first degree relatives of patients with schizophrenia.   In R.R. Fieve, D. Rosenthal, H. Brill (Eds.), *Genetic Research in Psychiatry.* Baltimore: Johns Hopkins University Press.

Tsuang, M.T., Winokur, G., & Crowe, R.R. (1980).   Morbidity risks of schizophrenia and affective disorders among first degree relatives of patients with schizoohrenia, mania, depression, and surgical conditions. *British Journal of Psychiatry, 137,* 497-504.

Tsuang, M.T., Woolson, R.F., Winokur, G., & Crowe, R.R. (1981). Stability of psychiatric diagnosis: Schizophrenia and affective disorders followed up over a 30- to 40- year period. *Archives of General Psychiatry, 38,* 535-539.

Tsuang, M.T., Faraone, S.V., & Day, M. (1988).   Schizophrenic disorders.   In A.M. Nicholi (Ed.), *The New Harvard Guide to Psychiatry.* Cambridge, MA: Belknap Press, pp. 259-295.

Tsuang, M.T., Tohen, M., & Murphy, J.M. (1988). Psychiatric epidemiology. In A.M. Nicholi (Ed.), *The New Harvard Guide to Psychiatry.* Cambridge, MA: Belknap Press, pp. 761-779.

Wallace, C.J., Nelson, C.J., Liberman, R.P., Aitchinson, Lukoff, Elder, et al. (1980).   A review and critique of social skills training with schizophenic patients.   *Schizophrenia Bulletin, 6,* 64-69.

Chapter 7
Mood Disorders

Each of the disorders in this group is characterized by a disturbance of mood: excessive elation, depression, or some combination of these. The disorder may reflect a single episode, periodic changes either in one direction or fluctuating between the two extremes, or a chronic pattern of affect disturbance. Because mood impacts on one's world view, these disorders tend to affect functional ability in global fashion.

Mood disorders are usually categorized either as depressive or bipolar. The bipolar disorders are those that fluctuate between mania and depression. It is rare to find an individual whose mood disorder is characterized only by manic episodes, i.e., episodes of extreme elation, although such a pattern is occasionally seen. The depressive disorders, however, are the most common of psychiatric disorders. These may be either ongoing chronic depressions, or periodic depressions caused by seasonal changes, stressful events, etc.

Figure 7-1
Mood Disorders, Severe to Moderate

Manic Episode	Bipolar Disorder	Major Depressive Episode
↓	↓	↓
Hypomanic Disorder	Cyclothymic	Dysthymic

This chapter will discuss the more severe mood disorders: manic episode, major depressive episode, and bipolar disorder, as well as the less severe but similar disorders: hypomanic disorder, dysthymic disorder, and cyclothymic disorder. The first group will be discussed in detail, the second, more briefly.

Manic Episode

These episodes are quite severe, usually of abrupt onset, and are characterized by major changes in attitude and behavior. Most prominent is an elevated or irritated mood, accompanied by a set of characteristic behaviors. These may include grandiosity, decreased need for sleep, talkativeness, flight of ideas, distractibility, increased activity, and excessive involvement in pleasureable activities with disregard for the consequences. For example, individuals experiencing a manic episode may spend money wildly, become involved in inappropriate sexual activities, and so on. Functioning is impaired in all spheres.

As with all psychiatric disorders, part of the diagnostic process is the exclusion of other possible disorders. If hallucinations and delusions are present, they must be accompanied by alterations in mood. In the face of such symptoms, schizophrenia, or other psychotic disorders must be ruled out. Although thought disorders may be present in individuals experiencing manic episodes, mood alterations are the most prominent feature of the symptom constellation. Organic factors such as intoxication must also be ruled out.

Other characteristics include emotional lability. The individual may be expansive and grandiose one minute, angry and hostile the next. There are frequent rapid shifts from mania to depression, and occasionally, the symptoms of the two appear together. Furthermore, the individual may be oblivious to his or her behavior, totally unaware that there is a problem.

According to Carlson and Goodwin (1973), three stages can be identified in manic episodes. During the first, prodromal stage, speech is pressured and tangential, mood happy, and hyperactivity evident. During the second stage, grandiosity and paranoia appear, and hyperactivity and pressured speech worsen. The third stage is characterized by incoherence, severe delusional content, and even more obvious hyperactivity. Disorientation to time and place is common. Recovery is evidenced by a reversal of stages. Not all patients reach stage three; some go only to the second and then reverse. Similarly, rate of progression is quite variable, from hours to days. In the prodromal phase, the individual might volunteer for a large number of projects at work, buy expensive presents for friends and family, and flit from topic to topic during conversation. This might progress to developing "new ideas" for work that are grandiose and strange, such as developing a space station to protect the country from invasion of aliens. The individual might sleep very little, talk and move constantly, and become extremely irritable. As the manic episode abates, symptoms will diminish.

Etiology and Incidence

Mania most often appears in individuals in their 20s, though it may have later onset. The most characteristic pattern of appearance is a rapid, abrupt onset. It is not clear precisely what causes the disorder, though family studies have established that there is a familial pattern. This pattern has appeared even when family members have been raised in different environments, and is thus a strong argument for some sort of genetic component to the disorder.

It has also been noted that manic disorders may follow severe psychosocial stressors (Dunner & Hall, 1980). For example, mania sometimes first appears following childbirth. Another documented cause of mania is head trauma (Shukla, Cook, Mukherjee, Godwin & Miller, 1987).

Pure manic episodes without accompanying depression are rare. Bipolar disorders (mania and depression in combination) are discussed below.

Prognosis

Prognosis for specific manic episodes is good. Duration of episodes is variable, although untreated they may last for a month or more. However, often there is a pattern of recurring episodes, meaning that without maintenance treatment, it is probable that the individual will have manic episodes on a periodic basis. In some individuals, the episodes follow a particular pattern, appearing each spring, for example, whereas in others they may appear unpredictably. In still others, there may be a single episode with no recurrence. Effective long-term treatment involves use of medication. In those individuals who are willing to take the drug as prescribed, it can be quite useful and can further improve prognosis. To prevent recurrence, however, it must be continued in maintenance doses for long periods. As will be discussed in Chapter 11, this presents a set of problems related to the potential for toxicity from the drug and the possible unwillingness of these individuals to follow the prescribed regimen. Use of maintenance doses of medication is problematic, given the nature of the disorder and the tendency to impulsive acts. As a manic episode develops, judgment and self-control are reduced, and the individual may stop taking the medication.

Because of the severity of manic episodes, hospitalization, often involuntary, is frequently warranted. Manic individuals demonstrate extremely poor judgment and must often be protected from a tendency to engage in illegal or imprudent acts or to abuse drugs.

Implications for Function and Treatment

As with schizophrenia, function is severely impaired. This is a defining characteristic of the disorder. Judgment is extremely poor and individuals tend to engage in acting out behaviors. For example, an individual may begin to gamble wildly, to take drugs or abuse alcohol, to argue with colleagues at work, or to become involved in promiscuous sexual activity. At the same time, impulsiveness and grandiosity interfere with vocational and social activities. There are changes in cognition and perception, although the exact reason for these changes is not well understood. Although motor skill does not change, hyperactivity is always present. It appears that there are some changes in CNS function that contribute to the characteristic symptom constellation (Klerman, 1988). Social impairment is marked (Dunner & Hall, 1980).

These individuals may be able to function quite normally between episodes. Depending on the frequency and duration of the manic periods, it is possible that they may hold jobs, have families, and carry on other activities most of the time. However, all these functions are impaired during episodes, often resulting in loss of job, family disruption, and so on. In those individuals who have reasonable levels of function between episodes, maintenance treatment with drugs, as well as family therapy to assist others to understand the disorder, may be quite effective.

When hospitalization is part of treatment, it is usually brief. The primary objective is to protect the individual from harm to self or others as a result of poor judgment and impulsivity. Once medications have begun to ameliorate the symptoms, hospitalization is no longer necessary.

Implications for Occupational Therapy

During the acute episode, an important role for the occupational therapist is monitoring behavior changes and providing a structured environment in which behavior can be managed. A typical manic patient might breeze into the clinic to begin "building a castle," switch to "creating a new Mona Lisa" after the first two nails are in place, then to making a leather coat after the first stroke of patient is on the canvas, etc. Clearly, limit setting is important. Signs of behavior change as medication is introduced are important to decision making about long term treatment.

Between episodes, the occupational therapist may assist the individual in coping with the possibility of a chronic illness. The individual needs to learn the signs of an impending episode to seek help. In addition, activity patterns may need to be examined to determine whether some stressful activities should be stopped or changed. Function in all areas of performance may be assessed to determine how stress can be managed, and how quality of life can be maximized.

For most individuals who have manic episodes, performance and skills are unimpaired between episodes. However, behavior during episodes may have long term consequences in terms of lost friends, family disputes, lost jobs, and financial difficulties. Clients need to learn how to avoid or manage these difficulties by altering lifestyle, monitoring symptoms, and getting family members involved. One woman learned that as soon as the lilacs bloomed each spring she would begin to have problems. Her husband learned to put away the credit cards, and she learned to go see her physician immediately.

Major Depressive Episode

The reverse of a manic episode, this disorder represents an episode of extreme depressed mood. To be given this diagnosis, an individual must exhibit depressed mood or loss of interest in pleasureable activities (anhedonia) for a period of at least 2 weeks. In addition, irritability, anhedonia, unintentional weight loss or gain, insomnia or hypersomnia (excessive sleeping), psychomotor agitation or retardation, fatigue, feelings of guilt or worthlessness, poor concentration, or frequent thoughts of death or suicidal ideation may occur. As with a manic episode, hallucinations, or delusions may be present, but the diagnosis is made only in the presence of depressed mood. In cases where psychotic symptoms appear without depressed mood, a diagnosis of schizophrenia or some other psychotic disorder would be considered. It is believed by some that "delusional depression" is more common in individuals with bipolar disorder (Weissman, Prusoff, & Merikangas, 1984).

This diagnosis will be made only in the absence of organic causes, and, more significantly, major depressive episode is distinguished from uncomplicated bereavement. In cases where an individual has recently lost a loved one, it would be considered normal to demonstrate the symptoms listed above. However, the therapist may need to identify a period beyond which major depressive episode as a diagnosis would be considered. This is somewhat problematic, as a wide range of opinion exists about the "normal" duration of bereavement.

With regard to diagnoses of depression, *DSM-III* and *DSM-III-R* mark significant departures from previous diagnostic listings. Most notably, they delete the prior distinction between endogenous and reactive depressions. In earlier editions, reactive depressions were described as those that had a clear cause, e.g., a significant loss or psychosocial stressor such as divorce or loss of a job. Endogenous depressions were thought to be those in which no clear and immediate cause for the depression was evident. It is now thought that this distinction is inaccurate as all depressions appear to have some identifiable precipitating event, even if it is temporally remote, and to have some identifiable biological component. This change is somewhat controversial, and not all researchers agree that there is no difference between the two disorders. However, the bulk of the evidence favors this conceptualization (Andreasen, Scheftner, Reich, Hirschfeld, Endicott, & Keller, 1986). Thus, the diagnostic distinctions among various kinds of depression are now made on the basis of specific symptoms and the pattern of appearance of depression in the individual's life.

There are two subcategories of major depressive episode. One is the melancholic type, which includes several symptoms in addition to those listed above. First, the individual must have had no personality disorder prior to the first depressive episode, must show good recovery between episodes, and good response to somatic treatments such as psychotropic medications or electroconvulsive therapy (ECT). These individuals display diurnal variation in degree of depression (typically worst in the morning), early morning wakening, and global loss of pleasure in activities. They tend to demonstrate depression so severe that it does not lift, even briefly, when some pleasant event occurs.

The other subcategory is a seasonal pattern (sometimes referred to as seasonal affective disorder, or SAD). In these cases, there is a specific pattern to depressive, and sometimes manic, episodes. Typically, these individuals become depressed in the fall and improve in the spring. This pattern must occur for several years before the SAD diagnosis will be made. If regular seasonal changes in life circumstances, such as regular winter unemployment or return to school in the fall, accompany the mood change, SAD will not usually be diagnosed. The most effective treatment for this type of depression is phototherapy, in which the individual is exposed to light for specified periods of time during the winter when natural daylight is less.

All of these depressive disorders may be accompanied by tearfulness, irritability, phobias, panic attacks, or excessive brooding. In addition, there may be somatic complaints. Major depressive episodes may occur in individuals of any age, and have somewhat different characteristics among different age groups. Children often have accompanying somatic complaints and psychomotor agitation, while adolescents often engage in substance abuse. Other antisocial behavior may appear, as well (Rutter, 1987). In elderly individuals, depression may present with symptoms of dementia.

One or more major depressive episodes in the absence of any manic or hypomanic episode will be called a major depression, either single episode or recurrent. Some individuals will have only one episode, while others have periodic episodes sometimes developing into bipolar disorder. Although most individuals with depressive disorders return to their prior levels of function between episodes, some have chronic form that is reflected by continuing low level depression and mild functional impairment.

Etiology and Incidence

Etiology of depression is poorly understood. As noted above, in earlier times a distinction was made between endogenous and reactive depressions. The assumption was that the former had biological causes, whereas the latter was the result of environmental factors. This distinction is not made as clearly any longer. It does appear that there is a biological component to depression, although there is some argument whether this is the cause or the result of the depressive episode. As with mania, there is a familial pattern to depression, arguing for at least some genetic component (Klerman, 1988). Other biological explanations focus on sensory changes (Amsterdam, Settle, Doty, Abelman, & Winokur, 1987), and on other CNS factors (Klerman, 1988). It appears, for instance, that depression is a common consequence of stroke, and that this type of depression is identical to other major depressive episodes (Lipsey, Spencer, Rabins, & Robinson, 1986).

It is also apparent, however, that depressive episodes correlate with psychosocial stressors. Chronic physical illness, substance abuse, and stressors such as divorce and childbirth have all been associated with depression.

There is a reasonable amount of support for the notion of stress as a risk/precipitant of depression in general (Hirschfeld & Cross, 1982), particularly for "undesirable" life events. However, life events alone do not cause depression. There seems to be an interaction between undesirable life events and indadequate coping responses in people who are biologically prone to depression (Hirshfeld & Cross, 1982). For example, individuals with biological predisposition to depression with high stress levels and poor personal resources (e.g., few social contacts) may be most likely to develop depression.

Psychosocial risk factors include early separation from parents (Roy, 1985), and marital status is also a factor (Hirschfeld & Cross, 1982), with separated and divorced individuals having greater risk for depression. Mothers at home with small children are also particularly subject to depression (Brown & Harris, 1978).

Other explanations of depression are behavioral (Lieberman & Raskin, 1971; Ferster, 1973), and cognitive (Blaney, 1977). It is possible that peculiar perceptions of the world, faulty interpretations of those perceptions, or an inadequate repertoire of responses may figure in the disorder. It is interesting to note that some research suggests that these individuals may have a too accurate picture of the world, to be unable to develop the small misperceptions that seem to protect nondepressed individuals from some of life's more unpleasant realities (Lewinsohn, Mischel, Chaplin, & Barton, 1980).

Major depressive episodes occur in between 15% and 30% of adults (Klerman, 1988). It is much more likely that an individual will have only major depressive episodes than only manic episodes. The disorder is much more common in women, as are all types of depression. The reasons for this difference are not known.

Prognosis

As with mania, prognosis for a specific depressive episode is generally good. Since Eysenck (1952) published his landmark work on the effectiveness of psychotherapy, it has been understood that some depressions will resolve within several months, with or without treatment. Some episodes, however, are chronic, persisting for years. Onset of an episode may be gradual over several days or weeks, or may be sudden. Some individuals may have one episode without recurrence, but a more typical pattern is recurring episodes, each of which resolves with return to premorbid function. The episodes may vary in frequency, or in the case of SAD, may be quite predictable in frequency, severity, and duration. It appears that depressions that are likely to improve without treatment do so within the first three months (Keller, Klerman, Lavori, Coryell, Endicott, & Taylor, 1984). More chronic patients had longer illness prior to treatment, other inpatient hospitalizations, intact marriages (a finding in conflict with the research reported above), low income, and other psychiatric disorders. Gonzalez, Lewinsohn, and Clark (1985) found family history to be a predictor of prognosis, that is, if relatives had the disorder, their course suggests what will happen to the individual.

Implications for Function and Treatment

Function in depressed individuals is greatly dependent on the severity of the episode. Some individuals may be able to continue nearly normal activity, whereas others may be totally unable to function.

At the level of specific skills, it is clear that cognition is almost always impaired. Concentration in particular is diminished, as is problem solving ability. Sensation is usually not affected, except in the presence of hallucinations, but psychomotor activity is often altered, either slowed or speeded. Social function is often poor, largely because of lethargy or anhedonia.

A great deal of research has examined the role of social skill in depression. It seems clear that individuals who later become depressed have poor interpersonal skills, including level and latency of activity, interpersonal range, and positive reactions (Libet & Lewinsohn, 1973). Silence and negative comments are typical (Howe & Hokanson, 1979). These problems occur in depressed adolescents as well (Puig-Antich, Lukens, Davies, Goetz, Brennan-Quattrock, & Todak, 1985). Although they may not cause the disorder, they may increase vulnerability (Vanger, 1987).

Poor social skills are problematic because of the reaction of others (Coyne, 1976). Those around the individual may become more hostile, anxious, and rejecting in response to the behavior of the depressed individual. Thus, the behavior of the depressed individual sets a cycle of disturbed interaction.

Another area of function likely to be impaired is avocation. Depressed individuals take little pleasure in activity, thus avoid hobbies, social activities, and other activities that they formerly enjoyed. They may be unable to concentrate enough to read or to enjoy television, movies, or other performances. They typically lack energy and motivation to engage in physical activities. Vocational function is also affected. Individuals who have creative jobs, or jobs that require high degrees of motivation such as sales, may find that they lack the energy and drive necessary to complete their required functions. In addition, cognitive and social impairment may interfere with their completion of tasks.

ADL and IADL may also be affected. In some individuals, this is primarily a matter of "not caring" about appearance or hygiene. In others, irritability, psychomotor retardation, lethargy, and loss of appetite may combine to result in greatly diminished function, sometimes to the extent that the individual takes no care at all of him or herself. He or she may not even get out of bed.

Coping skills of depressed individuals appear to be worse than those of non-depressed individuals (Billings, Cronkite, & Moos, 1983; Coyne, Aldwin, & Lazarus, 1981). Thus, their function may be impaired as they are unable to problem solve for everyday events. There has been some speculation that perceived lack of control over life events is an important factor, though this "learned helplessness" hypothesis is the subject of much controversy (Baucom, 1983).

Although depression is the most common of psychiatric diagnoses, it is also one of the most readily treatable. There is a vast array of psychotropic medications that may be quite useful in resolving a depressive episode. Many of them have undesirable side effects which make them unappealing over long periods, but they can shorten individual episodes and reduce their severity. Some of these medications may be taken on a maintenance basis to prevent recurrence and in general, medications to treat depression have been improved over the last 2 decades. For some individuals, electroconvulsive treatments (ECT) may be quite effective (Klerman, 1988). Generally speaking, when such treatment is applied, it is done for brief periods in the presence of specific sets of symptoms. This is quite unlike earlier forms of ECT that were given for a wide array of psychiatric disorders, and often for courses of dozens (or even hundreds) of treatments.

In addition, psychotherapy of various forms is felt to be helpful for depression. Cognitive therapies, for example, have grown in popularity as an intervention with depressed individuals. These therapies are based on the notion that depressed individuals inaccurately interpret events around them and that they can learn new and more helpful interpretations. Behavior modification and psychoanalysis, as well as a variety of group and family approaches, have all been reported to be successful with depressed individuals. Unfortunately, treatment efficacy is rather hard to establish since most depression does eventually resolve itself. Many evaluations focus on shortening individual episodes or preventing recurrences.

Suicide is a particular concern in the treatment of depression (Coryell & Winokur, 1982). The rate of suicide attempts is 30% for depressed persons (Klerman, 1988), i.e., almost 1 in 3 such individuals will make a serious gesture. Many depressed individuals contemplate suicide, and those who appear to have active suicidal intent may require hospitalization to prevent them from harming themselves (Klerman, 1988). The problem is complicated by the fact that some antidepressant medication can be lethal if abused, thus requiring careful monitoring, especially before it has had the opportunity to take effect in elevating mood, a process that may take several weeks.

Professionals who work with depressed individuals must be aware of the potential for suicide, note the presence of suicidal potential in these individuals, and take necessary precautions. It is helpful to ascertain by asking directly whether an individual is suicidal, and to determine whether a plan of action has been developed. This is ordinarily the responsibility of the individual directing treatment (team leader, psychiatrist, etc.), but other professionals should ascertain that this has been done. Individuals with a clear and feasible plan must be considered at high risk for suicide. In addition, individuals whose depression appears to resolve suddenly are considered high risks, as this may signify that they have reached a decision to act. Depressed individuals are at greatest risk during the period when the depression is just beginning to lift because they have increased energy to act on their suicidal wishes.

Precautions include careful monitoring, often in inpatient settings, and removal of means to cause death until the individual is clearly no longer actively suicidal. Although most suicide attempts are made with drugs and guns, other lethal substances and sharp implements should be guarded as well. There is a belief that some single car accidents are, in fact, suicide attempts, so it may be necessary to monitor driving, especially when accompanied by drinking, in these individuals.

Additional special note should be made about depression in children and youths. Although there is much debate on the subject, it appears that depression is quite common in children and adolescents (Cantwell, 1983). Symptoms may differ somewhat from those described for adults and usually reflect developmental stage. Anxiety, school refusal or school problems, and negative behavior are all common. As with adults, low self-esteem is common.

In children, school and social function are likely to be impaired. It may be difficult for the child to articulate the problem (or even to state that a problem exists). Teens often become sullen and withdrawn, behavior that should not be written off as "just a phase." Intervention must thus be sensitive to the age and stage of the individual child.

Implications for Occupational Therapy

Occupational therapists may focus on assisting the individual to find gratifying activities that improve self-esteem and increase motivation. In addition, activities that provide opportunities for self-expression are valuable since individuals who are depressed may be reluctant or unable to put their feelings into words. Art or other creative activities can provide a valuable outlet for such emotions. One very timid woman was asked to work on a woodworking project. After a few timid taps, she began to pound with the hammer, shouting with great enthusiasm "This is for my husband, this is for my boss, this is for the dog..." She was then better able to express her rage about feeling taken advantage of by those around her. Neville (1986) has suggested four major goals of treatment would be of value: re-engagement in valued activities, setting realistic goals for the future, re-establishment of routines and habits, and experiencing success and feelings of competence.

Since most individuals who are depressed do not lack the skills to do a variety of activities, motivation is often the key to improvement. These individuals may be extremely reluctant to engage in activity and sit passively throughout the day. Behavioral programs that reinforce desired behaviors can be valuable (Johnston, 1986). The exception with regard to skills is in the area of socializing. As has been mentioned, social skills training may be helpful to individuals who are depressed. In addition, activities that ensure positive reinforcement from others can be of great value. One woman spent a week baking cookies every day for the other patients. She thoroughly enjoyed their appreciation. At the end of the week, she was able to say, "Now I think I'll do something for *me*," and she began to knit a scarf for herself. She chose a bright cheery yellow that was in marked contrast to the drab browns and grays she had been wearing.

Bipolar Disorder

This disorder is characterized by fluctuations in mood, with episodes of both mania and depression. It is identified as mixed, manic, or depressed depending on the current or most recent episode. For example, someone with a history of both mania and depression who is currently depressed would be diagnosed as having bipolar disorder (BPD), depressed type. If there were currently rapid shifts it would be BPD, mixed. In most instances, this is a recurrent disorder, with some individuals having long periods between episodes, and others rapid alterations from mania to depression to relative normalcy. The episodes of mania or depression are those described above, although the duration of the depressive episodes may be less than 2 weeks.

Etiology and Incidence
There is a clear familial pattern in the appearance of bipolar disorder. In addition, the most effective treatment is lithium. Thus, there is strong evidence of a biological cause for the disorder.

The disorder is not uncommon, with estimates of its occurrence running at roughly 1% to 2% of the adult population of the United States (Klerman, 1988).

Prognosis

Although single manic or depressive episodes may resolve quickly, bipolar disorder is much more chronic than major depressive or manic episode (Coryell & Winokur, 1982). Each recurrence may further damage relationships, work performance, and so on, making functional problems cumulative. Education of the family is extremely important so that they understand the nature of the disorder and that the individual is not being intentionally disruptive. They can also be encouraged to help monitor symptoms, manage stress, and so on.

Implications for Function and Treatment

For specific episodes, functional decrements are the same as those described above for manic episodes and major depressive episodes. Between episodes, function may be quite normal. The individual will be able to work, engage in social and avocational activities, and perform self-care. This is particularly true for individuals who have long periods between exacerbations. However, as noted, some individuals have chronic problems, either because of the frequency of manic or depressive episodes or because of the consequences of the dysfunctional behavior in which they engage during the episodes.

Treatment of choice is medication. When taken as advised, lithium can minimize symptoms and prevent recurrences.

Implications for Occupational Therapy

Interventions for individual manic and depressed episodes in those with bipolar disorder are identical to those described in previous sections. Manic phase and depressed phase are no different for bipolar disorder than for major episodes. However, bipolar disorder tends to be chronic and intervention must address this as a concern.

Two important considerations apply. First, self-esteem and self-concept are likely to be damaged by both the chronic nature of the disorder and the enormous fluctuations in personality that characterize it. When an individual is sometimes withdrawn, sad, and lethargic and other times energetic and effervescent, it is difficult to form a clear picture of abilities or even desires. It is also difficult to feel good about one's performance when it is so unstable.

Medication may help the individual reach more even keel, but cannot repair the damage to self done by these mood swings. The occupational therapist must help the individual identify strengths, weaknesses, likes, and dislikes through exposure to a wide range of activities.

A second consideration is that needed skills may have been lost or may never have been acquired. One young mother had fluctuated between withdrawal from her two pre-school children and extreme irritability with them. She needed a good bit of training in parenting skills to resolve this and to begin to repair the damage done by her inconsistent and unpredictable behavior. This is fairly typical for individuals with long-standing bipolar disorder, particularly those who have not have adequate diagnosis and treatment.

Hypomanic Episode

Hypomanic episode is the diagnosis made when an individual shows signs similar to those in a manic episode, but when the symptoms are less severe and disabling. The distinction between major manic episode and hypomanic episode is one of degree. Although major episodes are quite striking, hypomanic episodes are less so, and are sometimes written off as excess energy. As with ADHD in children, the disorder is, to some extent, in the eye of the beholder. However, in many instances, judgment is impaired and irritability leads to fights with spouses, employees, etc. The individual may have rapid mood swings from euphoria to irritability, sleep less than usual, and start a wide variety of projects, none of which are finished. Hallucinations and delusions are not present, and the individual does not become disoriented to time and place.

Dysthymia (Depressive Neurosis)

This is a depressive disorder in which the individual has some symptoms of depression most of the time. Prior to *DSM-III*, the depressive neurosis label was used; *DSM-III* and *DSM-III-R* both use the term dysthymia. However, because depressive neurosis was such a common diagnosis prior to publication of *DSM-III*, the term remains in parentheses in the later manuals. For a diagnosis of dysthymia to be made, symptoms must be ongoing for at least 2 years, with periods of no more than 2 months at a time symptom-free. As hypomanic episode is a less severe form of manic episode, this is a less severe (though more chronic) form of major depression. The symptoms are milder, although they are more persistent. Dysthymia may precede a major depressive episode, leading to so-called "double depression." These are cases in which a major depressive episode is superimposed on a chronic moderate depression (Keller, Lavori, Endicott, Coryell, & Klerman, 1983). This is a particularly pernicious depression, with poor prognosis.

Dysthymia often coexists with other Axis I or Axis III disorders, in which case it is referred to as secondary. For example, many anorexics are depressed, as are some individuals with arthritis. In cases of secondary depression, the symptoms are less severe (Weissman, Pottenger, Kleber, Ruben, Williams, &

Thompson, 1977). Secondary depression occurs when there is a clear precipitating event but normal bounds of the mourning process have been passed. For example, death of a loved one, job loss or physical illness may lead to an ongoing secondary depression.

This is a very common disorder, although diagnosis may be difficult as the boundary between dysthymia and major depressive episode is not clear. Although *DSM-III-R* lists specific criteria, these characteristics are largely a matter of degree, and a moderate depression might be diagnosed by one practitioner as dysthymia, by another as major depressive episode. Dysthymia is notable primarily for its chronicity and for the absence of some of the more severe depressive symptoms, hallucinations and delusions, for example.

Function is generally impaired to a mild or moderate degree in individuals with dysthymia. Although they typically hold jobs, have social relationships and interests, these are not maintained at optimal levels because of the lethargy and lack of interest displayed by these individuals. Their constant depression wears on those around them and they may lose friends as a result of their inability to enjoy activities and to take pleasure in people. The chronicity of the disorder is a problem, as individuals tend to feel bad for long periods without relief.

Cyclothymia

This is a chronic disorder in which episodes of hypomania and depressed mood (but not major depressive disorder) are interspersed. It is a less severe form of bipolar disorder. For the diagnosis to be made, there must be at least a 2-year period during which the individual is symptom-free for no more than 2 months at a time. Some theorists believe that cyclothymia is simply a less severe form of bipolar disorder, and, in fact, the boundary between the two is indistinct. It is not unusual for cyclothymia to eventually develop into bipolar disorder.

By definition, cyclothymia is less severe than bipolar disorder, and this is evident in functional capacity. In fact, some individuals report that they are unusually productive during hypomanic episodes. Vocational function is, however, impaired during depressive periods. Social function is often impaired as the wide, unpredictable mood swings may cause difficulty for those around the individual. Substance abuse may become a problem as the individual attempts to deal with the depressive episodes or loses some capacity for good judgment during hypomanic episodes.

Implications for Occupational Therapy

For all the less severe mood disorders, hypomanic episode, dysthymia, and cyclothymia, principles discussed for the more severe disorders can be applied. Although the functional impact of these disorders is less, they can be very frustrating because of their chronicity. This alone can increase the depression and irritability that characterize the disorders. Thus, the individual may benefit from support in coping with chronic illness, education and information, and assistance in clarifying valued goals and activities.

Individuals who tend to be hypomanic often have difficulty with time management. They may be overcommitted and create interpersonal friction by being unable to meet their commitments. Effective use of time and realistic self-appraisal are important goals for occupational therapy.

Dysthymia presents an opposite problem although the consequences are somewhat similar. The individual has extremely low motivation that may be quite irritating to others. These individuals are the "Eeyores" of the world (Milne, 1947), constantly seeing the gloomy side of life (Munoz, personal communication, 1988). In their interactions with others, nothing is ever enough to help them feel loved and happy. These individuals need to discover activities that will be satisfying and motivating to them.

Cyclothymic disorder requires a combination of approaches, much like those suggested for bipolar disorder. Although the functional impairments are less extreme, their impact on self-esteem should not be minimized.

Figure 7-2
Mood Disorders

Disorder	Symptoms	Functional Deficits
Manic Episode	1. Abnormally elevated or irritable mood 2. Grandiosity 3. Decreased sleep 4. Distractibility, flight of ideas 5. Poor judgment 6. Impaired function 7. May be delusions or hallucinations	Work, social, leisure, cognitive psychological. May be mild-severe. Improves following/between episodes.
Major Depressive Episode	1. Depressed mood 2. Anhedonia 3. Appetite/weight change 4. Insomnia/hypersomnia 5. Lack of energy 6. Feelings of worhtlessness/guilt 7. Possible suicidal ideation	Work, social, leisure, cognitive psychological. May be mild-severe. Improves following/between episodes.

Figure 7-2 *continued*
Mood Disorders

Disorder	Symptoms	Functional Deficits
Bipolar Disorder	1. Recent alternating symptoms of both manic and major depressive episodes	As above
Hypomanic Episodes	1. Same as manic, but less severe	Same as manic but less severe
Dysthymia	1. Same as major depression, but less severe 2. Duration at least 2 year (1 for children)	Same as major depression, but less severe More chronic
Cyclothymia	1. Fluctuating hypomanic episodes and periods 2. Duration at least 2 years (1 for children) No more than 2 months symptom free.	Same as bipolar disorder, but less severe

References

Amsterdam, J.D., Settle, R.G., Doty, R.L., Abelman, E., & Winokur, A. (1987). Taste and smell perception in depression. *Biological Psychiatry, 22,* 1477-1481.

Andreasen, N.C., Scheftner, W., Reich, T., Hirschfeld, R.M.A., Endicott, J., & Keller, M.B. (1986). The validation of the concept of endogenous depression. *Archives of General Psychiatry, 43,* 246-251.

Baucom, D.H. (1983). Sex role identity and the decision to regain control among women: A learned helplessness investigation. *Journal of Personality and Social Psychology, 44,* 334-343.

Billings, A.G., Cronkite, R.C., & Moos, R.H. (1983). Social-environmental factors in unipolar depression: Comparisons of depressed patients and nondepressed controls. *Journal of Abnormal Psychology, 92,* 119-133.

Blaney, P.H. (1977). Contemporary theories of depression: Critique and comparison. *Journal of Abnormal Psychology, 86,* 203-223.

Brown, G. & Harris, T. (1978). *Social Origins of Depression: A Study of Psychiatric Disorders in Women.* New York: Free Press.

Cantwell, D.D. (1983). Depression in children: clinical picture and diagnostic criteria. P. Cantwell & G.A. Carlson (Eds.), *Affective Disorders in Childhood and Adolescence.* New York: Spectrum Publishers, pp. 3-18.

Carlson, G.A. & Goodwin, F.K. (1973). The stages of mania. *Archives of General Psychiatry, 28,* 221-228.

Coryell, W. & Winokur, G. (1982). Course and outcome. In E.S. Paykel (Ed.), *Handbook of Affective Disorders.* New York: Guilford Press, pp. 93-106.

Coyne, J.C., Aldwin, C., & Lazarus, R.S. (1981). Depression and coping in stressful episodes. *Journal of Abnormal Psychology, 90,* 439-447.

Coyne, J.C. (1976). Depression and the response of others. *Journal of Abnormal Psychology, 85,* 186-193.

Dunner, D.L. & Hall, K.S. (1980). Social adjustment and psychological precipitants in mania. In R. H. Belmaker and H. Van Praag (Eds.), *Mania: An Evolving Concept.* pp. 337-347.

Eysenck, H.J. (1952). The effects of psychotherapy: An evaluation. *Journal of Consulting Psychology, 16,* 219-324.

Ferster, C.B. (1973). A functional analysis of depression. *American Psychologist, 28,* 857-870.

Gonzalez, L.R., Lewinsohn, P.M., & Clarke, G.N. (1985). Longitudinal follow-up of unipolar depressives: An investigation of predictors of relapse. *Journal of Consulting and Clinical Psychology, 53,* 461-469.

Hirschfeld, R.M.A. & Cross, C.K. (1982). Epidemiology of affective disorders. *Archives of General Psychiatry, 39,* 35-46.

Howe, M.J. & Hokanson, J.E. (1979). Conversational and social responses to depressive interpersonal behavior. *Journal of Abnormal Psychology, 88,* 625-634.

Johnston, M.T. (1986). The use of cognitive-behavioral techniques with depressed patients in day treatment. *Depression: Assessment and Treatment Update.* Rockville, MD: American Occupational Therapy Association, pp. 49-61.

Keller, M.B., Klerman, G.L., Lavori, P.W., Coryell, W., Endicott, J., & Taylor, J. (1984). Long-term outcome of episodes of major depression. *Journal of the American Medical Association, 252,* 788-792.

Keller, M.B., Lavori, P.W., Endicott, J., Coryell, W., & Klerman, G.L. (1983). "Double depression": Two-year follow-up. *American Journal of Psychiatry, 140,* 689-694.

Klerman, G.L. (1988). Depression and related disorders of mood (affective disorders) In A. M. Nicholi (Ed.), *The New Harvard Guide to Psychiatry.* Cambridge, MA: Belknap Press, p. 309-336.

Lewinsohn, P.M., Mischel, W., Chaplin, W., Barton, R. (1980). Social competency and depression. The role of illusory self-perceptions. *Journal of Abnormal Psychology, 89,* 203-212.

Liberman, R.P. & Raskin, D.E. (1971). Depression: A behavioral formulation. *Archives of General Psychiatry, 24,* 515-523.

Libet, J.M. & Lewinson, P.M. (1973). Concept of social skill with special reference to the behavior of depressed persons. *Journal of Consulting and Clinical Psychology, 40,* 304-312.

Lipsey, J.R., Spencer, W.C., Rabins, P.V., & Robinson, R.G. (1986). Phenomenological comparison of poststroke depression and functional depression. *American Journal of Psychiatry, 143,* 527-529.

Milne, A.A. (1947). *The World of Pooh.* London: Linder.

Neville, A. (1986). Depression and the model of human occupation: Theory and research. *Depression: Assessment and Treatment Update.* Rockville, MD: American Occupational Therapy Association, pp. 14-21.

Puig-Antich, J., Lukens, E., Davies, M., Goetz, D., Brennan-Quattrock, J., & Todak, G. (1985). Psychosocial functioning in prepubertal major depressive disorders. *Archives of General Psychiatry, 42,* 500-507.

Roy, A. (1985). Early parental separation and adult depression. *Archives of General Psychiatry, 42,* 987-991.

Shukla, S., Cook, B.L., Mukherjee, S., Goodwin, C., & Miller, M.G. (1987). Mania following head trauma. *American Journal of Psychiatry, 144,* 93-95.

Weissman, M.M., Prusoff, B.A., & Merikangas, K.R. (1984). Is delusional depression related to bipolar disorder? *American Journal of Psychiatry, 141,* 892-893.

Weissman, M.M., Pottenger, M., Kleber, H., Ruben, H.L., Williams, D., & Thompson, W.D. (1977). Symptom patterns in primary and secondary depression. *Archives of General Psychiatry, 34,* 854-862.

Vanger, P. (1987). An assessment of social skills deficiencies in depression. *Comprehensive Psychiatry, 28,* 508-512.

Chapter 8
Anxiety Disorders
(Anxiety and Phobic Neuroses)

This group of disorders is characterized by the presence of anxiety, and, often, avoidance behavior. This section of the diagnostic list has undergone significant revision in *DSM-III* and *DSM-III-R*, with the addition of post-traumatic stress disorder (PTSD) and redefinition of other anxiety disorders.

Prior to publication of *DSM-III*, anxiety neurosis and phobic neurosis were the labels for these disorders. The name has been changed, but the earlier terminology remains in parentheses to help clarify the alteration.

Disorders in this category include panic disorder, agoraphobia, simple phobia, obsessive compulsive disorder, and post-traumatic stress disorder. (See Fig. 8-1)   Generalized anxiety disorder, a milder and less disabling disorder will be described only briefly since it is seen less often in occupational therapy settings. Occupational therapy intervention for all the anxiety disorders will be considered at the end of the chapter.

Figure 8-1
Anxiety Disorders

• Panic Disorder
• Agoraphobia
• Simple Phobia
• Post-Traumatic Stress Disorder

Panic Disorder

This diagnosis is made when the primary symptom is recurrent panic attacks. These may result in agoraphobia, an extreme fear of going into new or unfamiliar situations. Sometimes, however, panic disorder occurs in the absence of agoraphobia, and agoraphobia, as noted below, may occur in the absence of panic attacks.

Each panic attack is characterized by severe anxiety and feelings of panic, which may be accompanied by apprehension, shortness of breath, dizziness, nausea, chest pain, hot flashes, numbness, and fear of doing something uncontrolled. These attacks appear unpredictibly, particularly at first, and the individual may develop anxiety about the possibility of having a panic attack that is ongoing between attacks. Typically, the individual begins to associate these attacks with specific situations, which are then avoided, or begins to fear being anywhere that help might not be readily available, thus developing avoidance of any new situation (agoraphobia).

The attacks may be relatively frequent, several times a day, for example, or rare. Occasionally, the disorder is limited to one attack, or to a brief period during which the attacks occur, followed by a complete disappearance of symptoms. More typically there is a chronic pattern, with some periods of relative freedom from attacks, others during which the attacks become more frequent or more severe.

Etiology and Incidence

Panic disorder is quite common, but not well explained. It may occur in the presence of some form of depression, although the most common pattern is for depression to occur later (Coryell, Noyes, & Clancy, 1982), probably because the panic attacks can be so demoralizing. Panic disorder is often accompanied by a substance use disorder (possibly the result of attempts to self-sedate during panic attacks). It does appear that separation from family or disruption of important relationships during childhood is a predisposing factor.

Prognosis

Prognosis is variable, depending on severity, and on unknown and unpredictible factors. Some individuals, as noted, have time limited problems. Others have relatively chronic courses. It appears that suicide is common among individuals with a chronic course (Coryell et al. 1982) and that there is marked excess mortality from other causes, such as heart disease, over time.

Implications for Function and Treatment

Function is dependent on the severity of the disorder. In some individuals, functional impairment is minimal. Although they experience extreme discomfort during attacks, they may be relatively symptom-free between attacks, and may have long periods without problems. In other instances, function is severely impaired, particularly occupational and social function. Generally speaking ADL remains intact, although IADL may be impaired by unwillingness to go out. Some of these individuals, for example, experience panic attacks while driving, and, as a result, begin to refuse to drive.

Treatment is often a combination of antianxiety medications and behavior modification. Specifically, systematic desensitization has been found useful.

This involves pairing of increasingly anxiety provoking stimuli with relaxation methods to reduce the incidence of panic and to provide the individual with a sense of control of the symptoms (Nemiah, 1988).

Agoraphobia With or Without Panic Disorder

These individuals are afraid of having panic attacks or of being in unfamiliar situations, and therefore avoid going out. They are fearful of leaving a familiar environment, usually the house or even a specific room in the house. When the fear of panic attacks is based on prior experience of having the attacks, the diagnosis is agoraphobia with panic disorder. Some individuals fear panic attacks but have never had them. In this case, a diagnosis of agoraphobia without panic disorder would be made.

Etiology and Incidence

These can be very severe disorders, but their origin is not well understood. In most cases, prognosis is poor, as agoraphobia tends to represent a long term pattern of maladaptation. Although antianxiety medications and behavior modification have been employed with some degree of success, the disorder tends to be intractable.

Incidence is not well established (APA, 1987), as it is possible that some individuals needing treatment are unable to leave the house to go to a practitioners office or to a clinic. Agoraphobia with panic attacks is by far the more common of the two.

Implications for Function and Treatment

This disorder is extremely disabling. Although underlying skills (cognitive, sensory, motor) appear to be intact, performance is severely impaired. It should be noted that impact of the disorder on skills is not well understood. It is entirely possible, for example, that some sort of sensory change may contribute to the disorder, but this has not been well documented. What is clear is that these individuals have difficulty with most occupations. They cannot work because they fear leaving the house. Their social lives become quite circumscribed, and they are fearful of any activity that requires them to be in new situations. They may be able to maintain ADL, and those IADL functions that do not require them to go out. Their families may be involved in the condition as well. In one extreme case, the individual's husband reported that no one in the family was allowed to use the upstairs portion of the house, as this would precipitate a panic attack for the individual. Since the bedrooms were all upstairs, the family had to move beds into the living room. In some instances, the individual may be able to go out with one trusted companion, a friend or spouse.

Simple Phobia

These are phobias with accompanying panic attacks in the presence of a specific and limited object. In social phobia, for example, it is social situations that evoke the response. In simple phobias, stimulus to which the panic response has been attached. It may be a fear of snakes or of enclosed spaces, height, driving, flying, and so on. Unlike panic attack disorder, however, the source of the fear is identifiable.

Simple phobia diagnoses are not made unless the individual alters his or her behavior in some way as a result. For example, someone who is afraid of flying but does so regardless would not be diagnosed, whereas someone who avoided flying at all costs would be given a simple phobia diagnosis.

Etiology and Incidence

Phobias seem to develop through conditioning, i.e., an individual will have an experience with the stimulus that is anxiety provoking and then associate other similar experiences with the feeling of fear (Ost, 1985). A child who is frightened by a spider while playing outside may develop a feeling of panic in other circumstances where spiders are present. Alternatively, individuals may be taught their phobias or model on parent fears. In this case, a parent's fear of spiders might be conveyed to a child who then exhibits the fear as well. These phobias may persist for long periods. If they begin in adulthood, they will generally continue unless they are treated.

In all the anxiety states, neurotransmitters appear to be disturbed, particularly norepinephrine (Redmond & Huang, 1979). It is not clear whether this is the cause or the result of the anxiety.

Phobias are extremely common. Almost all individuals experience fear related to specific stimuli, and although most do not have panic attacks as a result, large numbers of people do.

Implications for Function and Treatment

Function is largely dependent on the nature of the feared stimulus. Social phobias may be relatively disabling as they lead people to avoid any situation in which new people will be present. However, many feared stimuli can readily be avoided without undue impact on the individual's life. Fear of snakes may be managed by avoiding most outdoor activity, a limitation that some individuals would not consider too great a hardship. Among the individuals most likely to seek treatment are those who have relatively late onset of symptoms that do interfere with function, i.e., a traveling salesman who develops fear of flying. Another particularly troubling phobia is school phobia, which is not uncommon in children. The phobia may develop as a result of a frightening or anxiety provoking experience at school, although in some instances it is unexplained. One child became sick every morning for weeks, until it was discovered she was afraid of the computer room at school, a small, windowless, rather dark space. Her symptoms abated when the computers were moved. In some cases the child refuses to go to school, in others he or she is too anxious to perform well while there.

Treatment usually involves some sort of behavior modification. Systematic desensitization has been found to be effective. Occasionally, antianxiety agents will be used, but this is not common, since the phobias tend to be circumscribed and self-limiting. Many individuals, in fact, find ways to alter their routines to avoid the feared stimulus entirely and never seek other treatment. The most effective treatment appears to be a combination of behavioral and physiological methods (e.g., biofeedback) (Ost, 1985). Cognitive approaches are less useful. Panic disorders appear responsive to antidepressant medications (Klein & Fink, 1962). Interestingly, Klein & Fink (1962) suggest that antianxiety agents are not useful. For more generalized anxiety states, the reverse appears to be true.

Obsessive Compulsive Disorder (Obsessive Compulsive Neurosis)

This is another disorder that was relabeled in *DSM-III*. Consistent with other diagnostic categories, the term neurosis was changed. The name remains in parentheses to assist practitioners in making the transition to the new terminology, and to help make comparisons easier in longitudinal (long term) follow-up research.

Obsessions are thoughts or ideas that are intrusive and anxiety provoking. Most common are obsessions with violence or contamination. The individual may recognize that these ideas are internally derived (not based on any external event), but is unable to control them and finds that the thoughts intrude while he or she is attempting to do something else (Nemiah, 1988).

Compulsions are repetitive, purposeful behaviors performed in response to an obsession with the goal of preventing the discomfort caused by the obsession. The activity is, however, either excessive or not realistically helpful in resolving the obsession. For example, someone with an obsession about contamination may engage in ritual handwashing or laundering of clothing, even though this in no way resolves the obsession.

Many obsessive compulsive individuals recognize the nature of the obsession and the futility of the compulsion, but experience great anxiety or tension when attempting to resist them. Over time, the individual may become increasingly unwilling to experience the anxiety and thus stop resisting the compulsion.

Depression, anxiety, and avoidance of anxiety provoking situations are commonly seen. Thus, in addition to engaging in ritual handwashing, an individual may begin to avoid unfamiliar situations that he or she views as providing further risk of contamination.

Etiology and Incidence

Etiology is not well understood, although some people believe this is learned behavior, whereas others believe that it is another manifestation of biologically generated anxiety. There is commonly a history of parental psychiatric disorder (Hollingsworth, Tanguay, Grossman, & Pabst, 1980). It most often occurs in young adults and may be precipitated by stressful events (Goodwin, Guze, & Robins, 1969).

Welner, Reich, Robins, Fishman, and Van Doren (1976) found several different presenting pictures for obsessive compulsive disorder among hospitalized patients. These ranged from uncomplicated obsessive compulsive disorder, sometimes with phobias or anxiety attacks, to obsessive compulsive disorder with depression (the most common picture), to obsessive compulsive disorder with psychosis or anorexia nervosa. This categorization is important to considerations of treatment, prognosis, and function.

The disorder in its most severe form is rare, but it appears that many individuals have mild forms of obsessive compulsive disorder.

Prognosis

Among children, obsessive compulsive disorder seems to be chronic (Hollingsworth, et al., 1980). For adults, the course is variable (Goodwin et al., 1969). Some do quite well, eventually returning to normal function. In others, it may be constant and chronic. In all individuals, the course of recovery is marked by exacerbations and remissions.

Implications for Function and Treatment

Depending on the compulsion, function may not be impaired or it may be severely impaired. Many individuals have some ritualistic, almost superstitious, behavior that is not disruptive (for example, wearing a particular set of clothing when taking a test, or checking the door lock exactly seven times before leaving home). However, in some cases, the compulsion may become the central focus of life (as in the case of an individual who must wash clothing 13 times before wearing it). Some of these individuals may be unable to maintain jobs, social relationships, or have any activity other than the compulsion. This is true despite the individual's recognition of the disabling nature of the compulsion.

Occupational performance is better among individuals with simple obsessive-compulsive disorders, as identified by Welner and colleagues (1976), and becomes worse as complications become more severe.

Obsessive compulsiveness may lead to social isolation, including a tendency to remain single (Goodwin et al., 1969). Many of the fears of these individuals do not tend to materialize, however. They are, for example, not likely to commit suicide, engage in criminal behavior, or become addicted to drugs even though these are common obsessional worries. Although the incidence of suicide and drug abuse is higher in these individuals than in the general population, neither is frequent.

Treatment involves the use of antianxiety drugs and behavior modification. There are no clearly documented effective treatments, however, and the disorder tends to be intractable.

Post-Traumatic Stress Disorder (PTSD)

The emergence of this disorder always follows an event that was a major life stress, one which must be more severe and unusual than those found in everyday life. For example, distress following a divorce would not be considered PTSD, whereas distress following a life-threatening fire might. The trauma may involve threat to one's life or the lives of one's family, destruction of home, victimization during a crime, or seeing someone else severely injured or killed. The trauma may be something that occurs only to the individual, as in cases of sexual or physical abuse in children, or to groups of individuals, e.g., holocaust survivors. In fact, PTSD was identified following the Vietnam War as a result of the large numbers of combat veterans who had extreme difficulty readapting to civilian life. It should be noted, however, that the syndrome certainly existed prior to this time, for example, as "shell shock" during World War I. World War II veterans who were prisoners of war showed signs of psychological distress long after the event (Tennant, Goulston, & Dent, 1986).

The trauma is usually accompanied by extreme feelings of terror and helplessness, and the primary characteristic of PTSD is a re-experiencing of both the event and these feelings that are recurrent and intrusive. The individual may have bad dreams, or find these feelings welling up at unpredictable times and in unpredictable places. As this occurs, the individual begins to avoid the situations that seem to stimulate it, or to develop a diminished ability to respond to the world as a mechanism for avoiding the unpleasant emotions.

Individuals who have this disorder have disturbed sleep, exaggerated startle reflexes, poor concentration, and extreme irritability often accompanied by aggression. It frequently occurs in conjunction with depression or anxiety.

Etiology and Incidence

Clearly, a traumatically stressful event is a necessary precondition to the emergence of this disorder. It is not clear, however, why some individuals are susceptible whereas others who have similar experiences may not develop PTSD. Obviously, not all war veterans develop PTSD, for example (although most report some change in outlook as a result of their experiences). There has been some speculation that individuals who develop the disorder had pre-existing psychopathology, but this is not well-established. It may emerge immediately after the trauma or after a period of months or years.

As the disorder has gained wider attention, the numbers of individuals diagnosed with PTSD has increased dramatically, and it is now considered relatively common.

Prognosis

Because this disorder has been identified so recently, prognosis is not well-known. It appears that some individuals have a relatively time limited disorder, whereas others develop chronic symptoms. By definition, it must last at least 1 month, but may persist for long periods. It appears, for example, that World War II prisoners of war showed high levels of depression 40 years after the war (Tennant et al., 1986).

Implications for Function and Treatment

Depending on the severity of the disorder, function may be minimally or severely impaired. Some individuals continue to hold jobs, to maintain social and avocational activities. It should be noted that a defining characteristic of PTSD is the avoidance of any stimulus that might cause the individual to remember the event. If it occurred in a place that is difficult to avoid, it may become quite disabling. Similarly, some individuals find that the re-experience of the event is frequent and that the accompanying fears are severe, leading to significant disability.

Effective treatment is not well understood, although it appears that group therapy, particularly where the individual can talk with others who have had similar experiences, may be of value. Antianxiety or antidepressant medication may be employed, although one of the concerns related to the disorder is the possible emergence of a substance abuse disorder as the individual seeks to relieve tension.

In children, where cases of sexual or physical abuse may be involved, remediation of the situation that led to the disorder is an important component of treatment. The abuser must be treated or the child removed from his or her presence, sometimes by removal from the family.

Implications for Occupational Therapy

Occupational therapists employ a variety of approaches in working with individuals with anxiety disorders. Several goals are prominent. First, an effort may be made to encourage relaxation, either by diverting attention or through relaxation training. The therapist might, for example, help the individual identify a pleasurable activity that requires attention (writing a poem, playing chess). This approach requires that the therapist be sensitive to the possibility that such activity could increase anxiety for some people.

Activities that require gross motor action to the point of fatigue may also promote relaxation, as will relaxation training. Once the client is relaxed, it may be possible to draw this to the individual's attention so he or she knows what it feels like.

Alternatively, it may be possible to use this relaxed state as a component of a systematic desensitization program. The relaxing activity can be paired with anxiety provoking stimuli until relaxation can be maintained.

A more controversial approach is flooding, where the individual is confronted repeatedly with the anxiety provoking stimulus until the anxiety response is exhausted.

For individuals with PTSD, opportunities to express emotion can be valuable. These individuals often benefit from talking with others who have had the experience, and from nonverbal expressive activities. One such client, a rape victim, progressed over time from drawing horrible monsters in stormy skies to drawing pleasant pastoral scenes. She found the activity both relaxing and cathartic.

As anxiety is resolved, attention must be paid to substituting new activities that are satisfying. An agoraphobic who is increasingly able to leave the house must find new and enjoyable ways to spend time formerly spent worrying. Individuals may need help re-establishing social ties, work activities, or leisure pursuits.

Generalized Anxiety Disorder

This disorder is characterized by a generalized state of anxiety or worry in the absence of specific reason to do so. The individual may worry excessively about the state of his or her health, or about finances, when there is no realistic basis for the concern. The diagnosis is not made if substance abuse or depression might cause the anxiety, although mild depressive symptoms may be present. This is usually a chronic disorder, although any functional impairment is mild. It is not unusual for secondary depression to occur, and individuals with this pair of disorders have a more severe and chronic course (Coryell & Winokur 1982).

Figure 8-2
Indicators of Anxiety Disorders

Disorder	Symptoms	Functional Deficits
Panic Disorder	1. Panic attacks 2. Four attacks within four weeks, or at least 1 month of anxiety about having an attack 3. Attacks include feelings of panic, sweating, dizziness, nausea, chest pain, intense fear	Work, leisure, ADL during attacks Fear of attack may impact on any function
Agoraphobia	1. Fear of being in situations in which escape is not possible 2. Avoidance of such situations	May be mild-severe If mild, often no impairment If severe, global impairment
Phobia	1. Intense fear of stimulus 2. Avoidance of stimulus	Dependent of specific stimulus. May limit any sphere.
Obsessive-Compulsive Disorder	1. Obsessions-intrusive ideas which may be distressing, cannot be suppressed, but are recognized as only ideas (i.e. *not* delusions) 2. Compulsions-repetitive purposeful actions intended to neutralize upsetting aspects of obsessions 3. Obsessions & compulsions	May be mild-severe Work, leisure, social ADL/IADL
Post-traumatic stress disorder (PTSD)	1. Experience outside the normal range of experience which is distressing 2. Recurrent distressing recollection/dreams about the event	May be mild-marked Most typically social, work, leisure

Figure 8-2 *continued*
Indicators of Anxiety Disorders

Disorder	Symptoms	Functional Deficits
	3. Avoidance of stimuli related to the event 4. Imsomnia, irritability 5. Physiological signs of fear 6. Minimum 1 month duration	

References

American Psychiatric Association (1987). *Diagnostic and Statistical Manual* 3rd ed., rev. Washington, DC.

Coryell, W., Noyes, R., & Clancy, J. (1982). Excess mortality in panic disorders. *Archives of General Pychiatry, 39,* 701-703.

Goodwin, E.W., Guze, S.B., & Robins, E. (1969). Follow-up studies in obsessional neurosis. *Archives of General Psychiatry, 20,* 182-187.

Hollingsworth, C.E., Tanguay, P.E., Grossman, L., & Pabst, P. (1980). Long-term outcome of obsessive-compulsive disorder in childhood. *American Academy of Child Psychiatry.*

Klein, E. & Fink, M. (1962). Psychiatric reaction patterns to imipramine. *American Journal of Psychistry, 119,* 432438.

Nemiah, J.C. (1988). Psychoneurotic disorders. In A.M. Nicholi (Ed.), *The New Harvard Guide to Psychiatry.* Cambridge, MA: Belknap Press, pp. 234-258.

Ost, L. (1985). Ways of acquiring phobias and outcome of behavioral treatment. *Behavioral Research and Therapy, 23,* 683-689.

Redmond, D.E., Jr. & Huang, Y.H. (1979). New evidence for a locus coeruleus-norepinephrine connection with anxiety. *Life Sciences, 25,* 2149-2162.

Tennant, C.C., Goulston, K.J., & Dent, O.F. (1986). The psychological effects of being a prisoner of war: Forty years after release. *American Journal of Psychiatry, 143,* 618-621.

Welner, A., Reich, T., Robins, E., Fishman, R., et al. (1976). Obsessive-Compulsive Neurosis: Record, Follow-Up, and Family Studies. I. In Patient record study. *Comprehensive Psychiatry, 17,* 527-539.

Chapter 9
Personality Disorders

These diagnoses are identified as Axis II labels according to the *DSM-III-R* schema. It may be recalled that this axis is specifically for disorders that characterize life-long patterns of adaptation; this is characteristic of personality disorders. In general they are less severe than Axis I diagnoses (with the exceptions of borderline, antisocial, and possibly schizotypal personality disorders), but they are also generally much longer lasting, with no periods of remission.

The personality disorders are also among the more controversial diagnoses for a number of reasons (Frances, 1980). First, they are less reliable than those on Axis I. To some extent this is because they represent exaggerations of traits evident in people without psychiatric disturbance. In addition, lifelong patterns are difficult to clearly establish in clinical settings. As Gunderson (1988) points out, "traits are identifiable as disorders only when they become so prominent and rigid as to cause dysfunction" (p. 337).

Some of the diagnostic criteria for these disorders have been described as arbitrary (Frances, 1980) and there is inconsistency about labeling of some disorders. For example, schizotypal personality is presumably a mild, nonpsychotic relative of schizophrenia and is found in the personality disorder section. Dysthymic disorder, which seems to be at a similar point on the affective disorder continuum (i.e., a mild, nonpsychotic relative of major depression), is an Axis I diagnosis.

Adding to the dilemma presented by these diagnoses, they are most often self-diagnosing, i.e., they are labeled only if the individual comes for help (or is sent by someone else). Many individuals who would otherwise be diagnosed never feel sufficiently bad or behave peculiarly enough to enter therapy. In some instances, it is the development of a coexisting Axis I disorder, most typically an affective or anxiety disorder, that brings these individuals into treatment (Gunderson, 1988). Once thought to be untreatable, personality disorders are now felt to be more tractable (Kernberg, 1975; Vaillant, 1977).

DSM-III-R identifies three clusters of personality disorders, which are grouped according to the overriding behavioral characteristics. The guide indicates that paranoid, schizoid, and schizotypal personality disorders (cluster A) are characterized by odd or peculiar behavior. Cluster B, antisocial, borderline, histrionic, and narcissistic personality disorders, present with flamboyant or dramatic behavior. The third category, cluster C, is for others that do not fit these two groups. The personality disorders will be grouped in this fashion for discussion here. It should be recognized, however, that the clusters have not been subjected to careful analysis and are somewhat subjective (Frances, 1980). Occupational therapy intervention will be discussed at the end of the chapter.

Figure 9-1
Personality Disorders

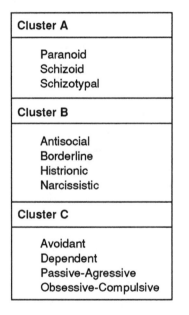

| Cluster A |
| Paranoid
Schizoid
Schizotypal |
| Cluster B |
| Antisocial
Borderline
Histrionic
Narcissistic |
| Cluster C |
| Avoidant
Dependent
Passive-Agressive
Obsessive-Compulsive |

Paranoid Personality Disorder

This disorder is identified by the individual's tendency to experience a sense of being threatened or persecuted. Friends and co-workers will be suspected of intending to harm the individual, and jealousy and suspicion characterize most relationships. This leads to withdrawn, suspicious, and frequently hostile behavior on the part of the individual (Gunderson, 1988). The personality disorder is less severe than paranoid schizophrenia, and is characterized more by misinterpretation of input rather than by outright delusions. For example, someone who has a paranoid personality disorder may interpret a minor reprimand from a boss as "he's never liked me; he wants to fire me; everyone here hates me." Someone with paranoid schizophrenia might interpret the same reprimand as part of a CIA/mafia plan to kill him.

Typically such individuals are argumentative, withdrawn, with little sense of humor and a "chip on their shoulders." They look for slights and frequently find them, tend to bear grudges, and may be litigious. They are hypercritical of others while accepting criticism of themselves poorly. They tend to be excessively self-sufficient and quite egocentric. One such individual had constant trouble at work because he routinely violated company rules, reasoning that they had been instituted only to harass him.

Etiology and Incidence

The etiology of this personality disorder is not clear, nor is its incidence. One explanation that has been advanced about its origin is that this is a learned pattern of behavior. Others feel that it is the result of some sort of CNS disturbance.

Implications for Function and Treatment

As can be imagined, this behavior pattern creates considerable difficulty for these individuals. The primary problem area is interpersonal relationships, both social and work. The suspiciousness and irritability of these individuals, coupled with their tendency to believe others are plotting against them, makes for troubled interactions, often resulting in lost jobs, divorce, and so on. In particular, relationships with authority figures tend to be problematic.

Other skills and functions remain largely intact. Motor and sensory skills, sensory integration, and cognition are, for the most part unaffected, except in those situations where the individual may believe he or she hears others talking about him or her. ADL, IADL, and work functions other than relationships with co-workers are maintained at acceptable levels, and these individuals may certainly maintain some leisure activities, mostly solitary. Treatment, through behavior modification, medication, education, or psychotherapy is not notably successful with these individuals. Their personality pattern tends to be stable, although some individuals can be taught how to interact more effectively with others.

Schizoid Personality Disorder

This is the oldest and best established of the personality disorder categories (Gunderson, 1988). It is defined by an absence or indifference to social activity and a restricted range of emotion. These are individuals often identified as "loners" who have no interest in friendships, appear aloof and withdrawn, and demonstrate little emotion. They may seem self-absorbed and vague. One such woman rarely spoke to co-workers, but often had what others described as a "peculiar smile" on her face.

Etiology and Incidence

The cause of schizoid personality disorder is not well established. As with paranoid personality, the major theories about its emergence are that it is a learned pattern of behavior and that it is due to some sort of CNS dysfunction. The latter explanation seems more likely. The disorder is more common in men and appears to occur in 2% of the population (Gunderson, 1988).

Implications for Function and Treatment

Again, the primary functional impairment is in the area of social relationships. Unlike paranoid personalities, however, these individuals tend to display little aggression, making work situations easier to maintain. Such people do well in jobs that require little social interaction (Gunderson, 1988). They have few social relationships, however, and rarely marry or have close friends. Akhtar (1987) identifies deficits in six areas of psychosocial functioning: self-concept, interpersonal relations, social adaptation, ethics, standards and ideals, love and sexuality, and cognitive style. Other skills and functions are unimpaired, meaning that these individuals are functional but lead lives restricted by the absence of meaningful friendships. The disorder persists throughout life, though some changes in specific characteristics may occur (e.g., the symptoms may come to more closely mirror narcissistic personality) (Akhtar, 1987).

When such individuals come into treatment, it is often because they are depressed about their isolation. Social skills training may provide a mechanism for helping them to establish relationships, although their interactions tend to remain stilted, awkward, or distant. Psychotherapy is sometimes attempted.

Schizotypal Personality Disorder

Schizotypal personalities have peculiar thought patterns, behaviors, and appearance. This may include bizarre fantasies, beliefs about special senses or powers, or odd patterns of speaking. Typically, odd perceptual experiences are present as well. Affect is either inappropriate or flat and social isolation is common. It is differentiated from schizophrenia largely by matter of degree; the symptoms are not severe enough to fit the criteria for schizophrenia, although the disorders are related (McGlashan, 1986). Such individuals are often described by neighbors as strange and as loners. If they have friends, their friends are often rather odd, too.

Etiology and Incidence

As with the other personality disorders in this cluster, etiology is unclear, but suspected to be the result of either CNS dysfunction or learning. Incidence is unknown, although the disorder is more common in family members of individuals who are schizophrenic (Gunderson, 1988).

Implications for Function and Treatment

It is unclear whether there is some dysfunction at the skill level. It is possible that CNS function is impaired, particularly ability to accurately process sensory input. Research has identified, for example, that smooth pursuit eye movement is impaired in these individuals (Siever, Coursey, Alterman, Buchsbaum, & Murphy, 1984). In addition, identification of characteristic cognitive-perceptual deficits have been helpful in making the diagnosis (Widiger, Frances, & Trull, 1987). These deficits may be the cause of some of the peculiar ideas held by these individuals.

At the performance level, function is distinctly impaired. Social function, in particular, is poor. Odd ideas held by these individuals make it difficult for others to understand them. The individual may avoid others because of discomfort in social situations and misperceive the social environment (Raulin & Henderson, 1987). Vocational function is impaired to the extent that social skills are required to do a job. As with schizoid personalities, these individuals may do best at jobs that require little social interaction. Actual work performance may also be poor, however, lending credence to the speculation that there is some underlying CNS or cognitive dysfunction. ADL performance is impaired; these individuals tend to be unkempt or to dress peculiarly.

Efforts at intervention are similar to those used for other disorders in this cluster, including medication, skill training, behavioral interventions, and verbal therapies.

Antisocial Personality

Of all the personality disorders, this is most likely to be brought to the attention of health-care professionals by someone other than the individual. The individual himself (this diagnosis is much more common in males) tends not to be concerned about the behaviors that create serious problems for others. This is also the personality disorder with the clearest diagnostic criteria (Reid, 1985), making its diagnosis more clear-cut than many of the others.

The diagnosis is made in individuals who are at least 18; prior to this a conduct disorder would be diagnosed, since antisocial personality is characterized by a lengthy pattern of behavior. The individual will have a pattern of antisocial behavior prior to age 15, e.g., truancy, fighting, cruelty to animals or people, stealing, and so on. In addition, this behavior will continue after age 15 with the addition of problems in work settings (loss of jobs, unemployment, absence from work), illegal activity, aggressiveness, impulsivity, lying, recklessness, and inability to function responsibly in significant relationships, e.g., parenting. A significant characteristic is the lack of remorse for any of these behaviors.

It is important to distinguish antisocial personality from other disorders, especially mania, since many of these behaviors will occur during manic episodes. The long-standing pattern of antisocial behavior makes it noticeably different, as does the absence of periods of remission. It should also be recognized that although these individuals are quite prone to criminal behavior, this is a unique characteristic among psychiatric diagnoses. There is a common misperception that individuals with psychiatric disorders are prone to criminal behavior. In reality this is untrue except for those with antisocial personality disorders (Tepelin, 1985).

Etiology and Incidence

Among the beliefs about the origin of antisocial personality is the theory that it is learned behavior, the result of overprotective or inconsistent parenting that does not allow the individual to learn that actions have consequences. Another theory is that cognitive and moral development are arrested at the 11-year-old age level, as these individuals show moral reasoning of this developmental level (Reid, 1985). There is also speculation about a biochemical etiology, supported by research showing neurotransmitter alterations, and by family research suggesting genetic links (Reid, 1985). None of the research is definitive. This disorder is more common in men, and is found in 2% to 3% of the general population (Gunderson, 1988).

Implications for Function and Treatment

There has been some speculation that antisocial individuals have sensory impairments. Some research suggests that a large percentage of the prison population shows signs of learning disabilities linked to sensory processing problems, but this remains unproven. Other research is conflicting: Gorenstein (1982) found evidence of deficits in cognitive tasks, specifically frontal lobe, however Hare's (1984) findings refute this.

Performance is impaired primarily in social and work spheres. ADL is intact with the exception of management of finances. Typically, money is a serious problem, with stealing a common solution. Social relationships are impaired by the lack of depth and conscience displayed by these individuals. They are unable, for example, to maintain monogamous relationships, and are unable to consider the feelings of others. Frances (1980) has suggested that this personality disorder would be better clarified if ability to experience loyalty, anxiety, and guilt were identified as factors to rule out the diagnosis, since prognosis is more favorable for those who have these emotions. One individual who was imprisoned for armed robbery and murder explained that he had to kill the security guard because the guard got in the way and therefore deserved to die. The prognosis for this individual, clearly, was poor.

In work situations, the belligerence and aggressiveness of these individuals is problematic. They may be quite able to perform the tasks required, but are not able to maintain acceptable relationships with co-workers and supervisors. They misinterpret some social situations, responding with excessive anxiety or anger (Sterling & Edelman, 1988). One man, during his short tenure on a construction job, routinely punched new employees just to "let them know who the real boss is."

In general, these individuals do not respond well to treatment. Those who have a diagnosis of depression as well do better (Woody, McLellan, Luborsky, & O'Brien, 1985), lending support to Frances' (1980) assertion that individuals who experience guilt represent a specific subset. Psychotherapy, inpatient, and outpatient milieu have all been shown to have some value. Milieu settings are usually structured to assure that actions do have consequences, thereby, at least theoretically, remediating previous faulty learning. Psychotropic medications do not seem beneficial (Reid, 1985).

Borderline Personality

This diagnosis has become increasingly common in the last decade and is a source of dispute since some do not believe it exists as a clinical entity. Recent research supports the validity of the diagnosis (Tarnopolsky & Berelowitz, 1987). It is probable that the increase is the result of changes in the diagnostic system, rather than an actual increase in numbers of individuals who fit this pattern. It is marked by instability of mood, relationships, and self-image, usually appearing during early adulthood. Relationships and affect tend to be unstable. Affect may also be inappropriate, in particular reflected by poor control of anger. Suicidal ideation and self-mutilation may also occur, and these individuals tend to be quite impulsive. They fear abandonment and have self-image problems characterized by uncertainty about sexual orientation, long term goals, or values. It is common to find depression or substance abuse coexisting in these individuals and to find a family history of alcoholism (Loranger & Tullis, 1985).

One borderline client had achieved a relatively stable work situation but found herself in great difficulty with her social life. Her boyfriends, all short term, routinely abandoned her and roommates moved out. Much of this was due to the extreme instability of her behavior toward them. She would be quite enamored and invested, bring daily gifts and write long letters about how close she felt to them. Within hours or days of this behavior she would write angry, spiteful letters, splatter their clothes with ink, and scream obscenities at them.

Etiology and Incidence

Since the disorder is more common in families in which there is a history of alcoholism (Loranger & Tullis, 1985), it is possible that a genetic component exists. However, it is also possible that borderline behaviors are learned from these dysfunctional relatives. The contribution of CNS dysfunction to the emergence of the disorder is not known. It occurs in 2% to 4% of the population (Gunderson, 1988).

Implications for Function and Treatment

As with other personality disorders, function seems to be impaired at the level of performance of self-care, work, and leisure tasks as opposed to motor, sensory, and other skills. There is no persuasive evidence to suggest abnormalities in sensory processing or other CNS function. However, vocational and social function are markedly impaired. Relationships tend to be unstable with these individuals fluctuating wildly between excessive involvement with devaluation of others. These relationship difficulties are the most consistent diagnostic criteria (Modestin, 1987). Difficulty handling anger and impulsiveness magnify interpersonal difficulties, as does a feeling of depersonalization that arises for many individuals with borderline personality disorder. Similar problems affect work. However, work problems are not solely the result of interpersonal difficulties. Since these individuals have problems identifying and maintaining a set of values and goals, they are unable to select and pursue career goals. Work history is unstable as they move from job to job or miss work because of substance abuse or suicide gestures.

ADL is unimpaired at a basic level, i.e., these individuals are able to dress, maintain hygiene, cook and eat, and so on. However, their impulsivity may lead them to ignore their ADL needs, to manage money poorly, drive recklessly, and so on. A particular issue with borderline personality is the tendency to "split," to see himself or herself and others as "all good" or "all bad" and to fluctuate rapidly between these poles (Goodman, 1983). These rapid shifts in attitude impact both on self-concept and on relationships with others.

Treatments recommended include long-term psychotherapy (Walding & Gunderson, 1987). In addition, a combination of short-term hospitalization, family education, and low dose neuroleptics seems effective (George, Nathan, Shulz, Ulrich, & Perel, 1986). Long-term milieu hospitalization has been reported effective as well (Tucker, Bauer, Wagner, Harlam, & Sher, 1987).

Prognosis is fair. In one study, 75% of borderline personality disorder patients followed for an average of 15 years were no longer diagnosable and showed functional improvement (Paris, Brown, & Nowlis, 1987). However, there was also a high risk for completed suicide.

Histrionic Personality Disorder

Histrionic personalities (formerly labeled hysterical personalities) demonstrate excessive emotionality or theatricality and attention-seeking behavior. They tend to need a great deal of approval or reassurance, which they may seek by being sexually seductive, excessively concerned with physical attractiveness, and attempting to be the center of attention in all situations. Self-centeredness is extreme, and emotions are exaggerated. At the same time, emotions shift rapidly and are quite shallow. These individuals have low thresholds for frustration and are unable to delay gratification. It has been suggested that they fear being unloveable and seek attention to reassure themselves that this is not so (Gunderson, 1988).

Etiology and Incidence
This is almost certainly a learned pattern of behavior. Problem relationships with family members have been implicated as fostering the insecurity that is notable in these individuals. Prevalence is unknown.

Implications for Function and Treatment
Histrionic personality disorder does not seem to impair cognitive, sensory and perceptual skills. Rather, this disorder impairs function at the performance level, specifically in social situations. Friendships are superficial, and focused on the individual. They are unable to respond with genuine emotion to the needs of others. They romanticize relationships and respond with excessive disappointment to disagreements. One such young woman arrived at work to announce loudly and tearfully that she would have to "end it all" because her boyfriend had to cancel a date because he had the flu.

Such individuals may be unpleasant to be around in work situations, but they are typically able to function at work. They may, however, have problems with co-workers or supervisors and are prone to quit unpredictably when they become bored. ADL is usually not impaired; in fact, such individuals may spend a great deal of time on hygiene and grooming to be attractive to others. They often dress quite seductively, then act puzzled when others respond to the apparent seduction.

Some of these individuals are able to learn new behaviors, often through behavior modification, and to develop insight into their behavior through psychotherapy. Making the changes tends to be quite difficult, however, and most often, when they seek treatment, these individuals want a "quick fix" for an immediate crisis rather than any major change in their attitudes or behaviors. One woman came into therapy because her father had "disowned" her and she was "now an orphan." It turned out he had stopped her allowance when, at age 25, she got a job. Her wish for therapy was that the therapist call her father and tell him to resume the allowance.

Implications for Occupational Therapy

A useful focus for occupational therapy is activity that builds self-esteem. Experiences of success and the appreciation of others may help convince these individuals of their worth. The insecurity tends to be so deep, however, that it is quite problematic to provide them with all the reassurance they need.

Narcissistic Personality Disorder

Grandiosity is the defining feature of this disorder. This is accompanied by a lack of empathy for others and excessive sensitivity to attitudes of others toward self. These individuals identify themselves as special, exaggerate accomplishments and feel entitled to recognition and special attention. However, these feelings fluctuate with feelings of insecurity and unworthiness. Self-esteem is poor but is masked by expressions of superiority. There is focus on fantasies of power and success, accompanied by feelings of envy for those who have accomplished more.

Etiology and Incidence

Like histrionic personality disorder, this appears to be a learned pattern of adaptation, the result of disordered family life. These individuals may get conflicting messages from parents, feel undervalued, and, as a result, come to undervalue themselves. At the same time, their grandiosity is an attempt to win approval that may not have been forthcoming in their homes. Incidence is unknown.

It is poorly understood because it is one of the less well researched personality disorders (Gunderson, 1988).

Implications for Function and Treatment

This disorder does not appear to cause dysfunction at the skill level. Sensation, cognition, and motor function are intact. Primary dysfunction is noted in interpersonal relationships. These individuals are self-centered and unable to display empathy for others, making friendships difficult for them. This pattern is also problematic in work situations where relationships with supervisors may be difficult. In some situations, vocational performance may be unusually good as the individual strives for great success, whereas in others performance is poor as the individual becomes resentful of expectations of others. One man had a long work history of jobs that lasted 6 months at a stretch. As each began he had "great new plans to save the company." As each ended, he excoriated his co-workers for failing to recognize his "genius." ADL is usually unimpaired, although money management may become an issue. In an attempt to impress others, these individuals may spend to excess. When these individuals present for treatment, it is usually for depression as a result of their social isolation. It is rare that they are able to develop insight or to change behaviors, as they tend to blame others for their problems and to be impatient with the therapeutic process. In most instances, the depression rather than the personality disorder is the focus of treatment.

Avoidant Personality Disorder

Social discomfort and avoidance of interpersonal relationships is the primary characteristic of this disorder. These individuals fear that others will disapprove of them, and, as a result, avoid interaction (Frances & Widiger, 1986).

Etiology and Incidence
This is probably a learned pattern of behavior. It appears to result from poor early experiences with relationships. Incidence in unknown.

Implications for Function and Treatment
Most function is intact in these individuals at the level of performance, but affected by the inability to form relationships. These individuals work, and care for themselves, but have emotionally and socially restricted lives. Skills are unimpaired, with the exception of social skills. Even in this sphere, superficial relationships may be adequate. One client was a university professor who managed brief casual interactions with students, as well as the more formalized classroom relationships. His personal life, however, was barren of friends or close family ties

As with narcissistic personality disorder, these individuals often seek treatment as a result of depression. Treatment may focus on insight or behavior change, or a combination of the two. Unlike individuals with narcissistic personality disorders, these individuals may be able to make a committment to treatment, and to benefit from it.

Dependent Personality Disorder

Avoidant personalities avoid relationships, dependent personalities feel they cannot survive without them. They are dependent and submissive in an attempt to win approval and to avoid abandonment. They have diffficulty making decisions and look to others to tell them what to do. As a result, they are unable to successfully initiate activity. They fear being alone.

Etiology and Incidence

As with other disorders in this cluster, this is probably a learned behavioral pattern. Prevalence is not established, but it is probably common (Gunderson, 1988).

Implications for Function and Treatment

Performance is intact in these individuals, although they are limited by their need for approval and advice from others. In social situations, friends are granted excessive control, and in work situations they are unable to progress because of their inability to take initiative and function independently. One woman refused to buy new clothes without approval from her husband and her mother.

Individuals with dependent personality disorder often come into treatment as a result of depression or anxiety that results from fears of abandonment. In many instances, the abandonment is real, as dependent personalities are quite draining to others. This is a difficult disorder to treat, although psychotherapy and behavior modification can be of value in some instances.

Obsessive Compulsive Personality Disorder

This is potentially the most disabling of the cluster C personality disorders, as these individuals are perfectionistic, rigid, and engage in ritualistic behavior. They never feel they have done well enough, and they focus on minor details, wasting time that could be better spent. Decision making is difficult as these individuals are unable to evaluate choices and act. They are judgmental and moralistic, often quite stingy and have difficulty expressing warmth. It has been theorized that these individuals have an extreme need for acceptance, causing conflicts about autonomy (Salzman, 1980).

Etiology and Incidence

Etiology is not well-established. It is possible that the same CNS dysfunction that seems to contribute to obsessive compulsive disorder may also contribute to obsessive compulsive personality disorder, making it simply a less severe manifestation of the same problem. It is also possible that this is a learned problem or evidence of developmental delay, as many young children demonstrate obsessive compulsive behavior (e.g., "step on a crack, break your mother's back" leads to careful avoidance of cracks in the sidewalk in many 8-year-olds). Most children outgrow these compulsions rather quickly, but there is speculation that these individuals do not for some reason. Prevalence is about 2% in the adult population (Gunderson, 1988).

Implications for Function and Treatment

Primary impairments that result from this disorder are social and vocational. The rigidity and moralistic nature of these individuals makes it difficult for them to form warm relationships. Their perfectionism, difficulty making decisions, and inability to use time well make work performance less than optimal. Task completion, in particular, is problematic. One individual, a bookkeeper, was unable to complete any page that had an erasure, and as a result was unable to complete assigned tasks.

Treatment of the personality disorder is difficult, although most often intervention focuses on depression. These individuals tend to be aware of their behavior and the problems it causes. In some instances, this leads to considerable depression or anxiety.

Passive Aggressive Personality Disorder

These individuals develop a pattern of passive resistance in work and social relationships. They procrastinate, are irritable when asked to complete tasks, and appear to deliberately avoid things they do not wish to do. They "forget," obstruct, and criticize others. At the same time, they believe they are doing well but that others do not appreciate them.

Etiology and Incidence

This is another personality disorder that seems to be a learned pattern of adaptation. Because this diagnosis relies on one trait, it is highly unreliable (Gunderson, 1988). In particular, it is possible to see the behavior exhibited in specific situations or at specific times, thus failing to meet the personality disorder criterion of being a lifelong behavioral pattern. It is not unusual, for example, for an individual to display passive aggressive behavior in a situation in which he or she feels powerless, perhaps work. This would not by itself qualify one for the diagnosis. Although the diagnosis is rare, passive aggressive behavior is common.

Implications for Function and Treatment

Skills are unimpaired, as is ADL, but work and social performance are dysfunctional. This is the result of the resistance to demands and resentment of others. Social relationships are very poor as these individuals can be quite unpleasant. They may, for example give backhanded compliments, e.g., "You look nice today, for a change," or be quite negative and oppositional, e.g., finding fault with every suggestion for an evening's entertainment. Since all this behavior is accompanied by a smile, it can be quite frustrating to others, who get angry but are not sure why. Thus, individuals with a passive aggressive behavior pattern tend to have few long term or close friends.

As with other personality disorders, these individuals often enter treatment for a secondary depression. Insight into their behavior is usually limited, though they are capable of gaining better understanding of their effect on others. Changing the behavior is very problematic, however, because they are often unaware of the impact of particular behavior at the moment. They often express puzzlement about the obvious irritation of others. Behavior modification can have some value, though it is unlikely that the underlying tendency will be altered.

Implications for Occupational Therapy

Although the manifestations of various personality disorders differ, the underlying issues are similar: inaccurate perceptions of self and others; inadequate social skills; poorly developed personal values and goals; and poor self-esteem. For some, particularly the cluster A disorders, inaccurate perceptions extend to many situations. This cluster may also be characterized by subtle neurological deficits in addition to the faulty learning that has been implicated as an etiological factor for all the personality disorders.

Because of the commonality of issues, some general approaches may be taken by the occupational therapist. Opportunities for group interaction with clear, consistent feedback may be quite valuable. A variety of group or cooperative activities may be helpful, from planning a social event to social skills training. A particular goal for feedback is interpreting accurately what others say and developing empathy. It is fairly characteristic that individuals with personality disorders show little regard for the feelings of others, and they must learn to make an active effort to do so. One histrionic client, a young female college student, was quite astonished to learn that other females resented her tendency to flirt with their boyfriends. It had never occurred to her to consider their feelings, even though she felt unhappy about her lack of girlfriends.

Realistic appraisal of self is similarly problematic. Provisions of a range of activities may be useful as a mechanism for exploration and for learning strengths and weaknesses. Both successes and failures must be analyzed. This not only enhances self-awareness, but also is a way to explore values and goals. It is hoped that enough successes are experienced to enhance self-esteem as well.

The three clusters present with somewhat differing characteristics that must also be addressed. Cluster A personality disorders, because of the suspected neurological component, may respond to sensory integrative/ sensorimotor interventions. Cluster B, because of the probability that they reflect deficits in early learning, may be appropriate for behavioral approaches. For example, a work experience might be structured in the clinic with reinforcement for desired behaviors.

Cluster C personality disorders may be particularly amenable to social skills training since this is the predominant deficit for these individuals.

All the personality disorders are, however, somewhat intractable. Although change is possible, it requires considerable motivation which is often lacking in these individuals. Even those who are motivated may find change frightening and will certainly find ingrained habits hard to alter.

Figure 9-2
Indicators of Personality Disorder

Disorder	Symptoms	Functional Deficits
CLUSTER A Paranoid Personality Disorder	1. Tendency to suspect others, to interpret their actions as hostile	Work, leisure, social
Schizoid	1. Lack of interest in social relationships 2. Restricted emotional range	Work, leisure, social
Schizotypal	1. Poor relationships 2. Restricted emotional range 3. Odd perceptual experiences 4. Odd appearance, speech 5. Inappropriate affect	Work, leisure, social, ADL/IADL
CLUSTER B Antisocial	1. At least 18 years old 2. Previous conduct disorder	Work, leisure, social, IADL (esp. financial)

Figure 9-2 *continued*
Indicators of Personality Disorder

Disorder	Symptoms	Functional Deficits
	3. At least four types of antisocial behavior (theft, lying, child abuse, etc.) which occur in a persistent pattern 4. Lacks remorse/guilt 5. Inability to sustain relationships	
Borderline	1. Relationships fluctuate between intense involvement and devaluation 2. Impulsiveness, instability 3. Lack of control of anger 4. Suicide gestures or self mutilation	Work, leisure, social, ADL/IADL
Histrionic	1. Excessive concern with appearance; seductive 2. Excessive need for praise reassurance 3. Self-centered; lack of empathy for others 4. Exaggerated expression of emotion, with rapid mood shifts, shallow emotion 5. Need for constant attention	Work, leisure, social,
CLUSTER C Avoidant	1. Discomfort with social relationships 2. Avoidance of social relationships and activities	Social, possibly work and leisure

Figure 9-2 *continued*
Indicators of Personality Disorder

Disorder	Symptoms	Functional Deficits
Dependent	1. Excessive dependence and submissive behavior 2. Fear of abandonment 3. Easily hurt by criticism	Social, possibly work and leisure
Obsessive - Compulsive	1. Perfectionism 2. Indecisiveness 3. Preoccupation with detail 4. Lack of generosity, empathy 5. Excessive moralism, conscientiousness	Work, leisure, social
Passive - Aggressive	1. Resistance to demands for ordinary/normal performance 2. Procrastination 3. Irritability or forgetfulness when asked to do something 4. Resentfulness and obstructionism	Social, work, sometimes leisure

References

Akhtar, S. (1987). Schizoid personality disorder: A synthesis of developmental, dynamic, and descriptive features. *American Journal of Psychotherapy, 41,* 449-518.

Frances, A. (1980). The *DSM-III* personality disorders section: A commentary. *American Journal of Psychiatry, 137,* 1050-1054.

Frances, A. & Widiger, T. (1986). Avoidant personality. In B. Karasu (Ed.), *Treatment of Psychiatric Disorders.* Washington, D.C.: American Psychiatric Press.

Goodman, G.B. (1983). Occupational therapy treatment: Interventions with borderline patients. *Occupational Therapy in Mental Health, 3*(3), 19-32.

Gorenstein, E.E. (1982). Frontal lobe functions in psychopath. *Journal of Abnormal Psychology, 91,* 368-379.

Gunderson, J.C. (1988). Personality disorders. In A.M. Nicholi (Ed.), *The New Harvard Guide to Psychiatry.* Cambridge, MA: Belknap Press, pp. 337-357.

Hare, R.D. (1984). Performance of psychopaths on cognitive tasks related to frontal lobe function. *Journal of Abnormal Psychology, 93,* 133-140.

Kernberg, O. (1975). *Borderline Conditions and Pathological Narcissism.* New York: Aronson.

Loranger, A.W. & Tullis, E.H. (1985). Family history of alcoholism in borderline personality disorder. *Archives of General Psychiatry, 42,* 153-157.

McGlashan, T.H. (1986). Schizotypal personality disorder. *Archives of General Psychiatry, 43,* 329-334.

Modestin, J. (1987). Quality of interpersonal relationships: The most characteristic *DSM-III* BPD criterion. *Comprehensive Psychiatry, 28,* 397-402.

Paris, J., Brown, R., & Nowlis, D. (1987). Long-term follow-up of borderline patients in a general hospital. *Comprehensive Psychiatry, 28,* 530-535.

Raulin, M.J. & Henderson, C.A. (1987). Perception of implicit relationships between personality traits by schizotypic college subjects. A pilot study. *Journal of Clinical Psychology, 43,* 463-467.

Reid, W.H. (1985). The antisocial personality: A review. *Hospital and Community Psychiatry,* 36, 831-837.

Salzman, L. (1980). *Psychotherapy of the Obsessive Personality.* New York: Aronson.

Sterling, S. & Edelman, R.J. (1988). Reactions to anger and anxiety-provoking events: Psychopathic and nonpsychopathic groups compared. *Journal of Clincial Psychology, 44,* 96-100.

Siever, L.J., Coursey, D., Alterman, I.S., Buchsbaum, M.S., & Murphy, D.L. (1984). Impaired smooth pursuit eye movement: vulnerability marker for schizotypal personality in a normal volunteer population. *American Journal of Psychiatry, 141,* 1560-1565.

Tarnopolsky, A. & Berelowitz, M. (1987). Borderline personality: A review of recent research. *British Journal of Psychiatry, 151,* 724-734.

Teplin, L.A. (1985). The criminality of the mentally ill: a dangerous misconception. *American Journal of Psychiatry, 142,* 593-599.

Tucker, L., Bauer, S.F., Wagner, S., Harlam, D., & Sher, I. (1987). Long-term hospital treatment of borderline patients: A descriptive outcome study. *American Journal of Psychiatry, 144,* 1443-1448.

Vaillant, G.E. (1977). *Adaptation to Life.* Boston: Little, Brown.

Walding, R. & Gunderson, J. (1987). *Effective Psychotherapy with Borderline Patents.* New York: Macmillan

Widiger, T.A., Frances, A., & Trill, T.J. (1987). A psychometric analysis of the social-interpersonal and cognitive-perceptaul items for the schizotypal personality disorder. *Archives of General Psychiatry, 44,* 741-745.

Woody, G.E., McLellan, A.T., Luborsky, L., & O'Brien, C.P. (1985). Sociopathy and psychotherapy outcome. *Archives of General Psychiatry, 42,* 1081-1086.

Chapter 10
Other Disorders

There are a large number of disorders that have not been discussed in previous chapters either because they are uncommon or because they are seen infrequently by occupational therapists. However, it is useful to be familiar with their fundamental characteristics as they do appear, not only in mental health facilities, but also in other health care settings.

First, it is helpful to know that all the categories of diagnosis previously discussed include a "not otherwise specified" (NOS) label. These may be considered residual categories, used in situations in which the individual fits most but not all of the criteria, or when presentation is in some way atypical. There are also labels for deferred diagnoses, or for those situations in which there is an Axis I but not Axis II disorder, or Axis II without Axis I. For example, an individual may present with clear symptoms of schizophrenia, but not fit precisely in one of the subgroups. In this case, NOS would be applied. If someone is diagnosed as dysthymic, the therapist might defer Axis II diagnosis rather than say none, if he or she is uncertain whether or not a personality disorder coexists.

In addition, many of the categories have subheadings that allow for greater specificity where it is possible to make more concrete identification of the symptom constellation. For example, panic disorder may be with or without agoraphobia, major depression may be identified as single episode or recurrent, and so on. These subheadings, which can be seen in the appendix, provide clarifying information to assist with treatment decisions.

There are also several groups of disorders that are useful to recognize, as they may well be represented in psychiatric populations. Because the disorders described in this section are not frequently seen in occupational therapy, description of each will be brief. When individuals with these disorders are referred to occupational therapy, treatment must be based on a theoretical framework that can guide assessment and intervention.

Figure 10-1
Other Psychiatric Syndromes/Disorders

```
"Not Otherwise Specified"
Gender Identity Disorders
Tic Disorders
Elimination Disorders
Speech Disorders
Other Disorders of Infancy, Childhood,
    and Adolescence
Somatoform Disorders
Dissociative Disorders
Sexual Disorders
Sleep Disorders
Factitious Disorders
Impulse Disorders not Elsewhere Classified
Adjustment Disorders
V Codes
```

Gender Identity Disorders

These disorders reflect conflict between assigned sex and gender identity. Specifically, they reflect extreme discomfort with assignment as male or female, and a conviction that the individual should be the other sex. In the most extreme form, this is reflected as transsexualism, in which the individual may simply choose to live as if the other sex, and possibly to have hormonal and surgical treatment to allow reassignment. Transsexualism is quite rare, and is not to be confused with tomboyishness in girls, "feminine" behavior in boys, or anxiety about living up to sex role expectations. It reflects a profound belief that the individual was born in the wrong body. This belief is most often present in childhood, where the child is distressed about his or her sex, insistence that he or she is really the opposite sex.

The cause of these disorders is unknown, with speculation ranging from prenatal hormonal exposure to genetic flaws to learned behaviors. Research is inconclusive about the roots of the problem, but it does seem to appear early in childhood in most cases.

Treatment provides two primary alternatives (Edelman, 1986). One involves sex reassignment, including hormonal treatment and sometimes surgery, to make the body more consistent with gender assumed by the individual. This approach also requires extensive therapy to work through psychological difficulties associated with this kind of dramatic change and to provide training about appropriate gender behavior. The other treatment is to help the individual feel more comfortable with existing sex assignment. This second alternative is facilitated through skill training, behavior therapy, psychotherapy, and occupational therapy to teach appropriate sex role behavior (Khanna, Desai, & Channabasavanna, 1987). Both approaches are successful with some individuals (Edelman, 1986; Khanna et al, 1987).

There is a group of individuals who present the greatest treatment problem. This is the group who choose not to have surgery, but are uncertain about the decision (Kockott & Fahrner, 1987). These individuals have the poorest long term adaptation and are most likely to need psychotherapy. They are typically older and have made an effort to live within their biological sex role by marrying, having children, and so on.

Tic Disorders

These include Tourette's syndrome, chronic motor or vocal tic disorder, and transient tic disorder. Tics are involuntary, sudden, stereotyped motor or vocal movements. They may be simple, as an involuntary eye-blinking or neck jerking movement, or grunting or snorting. Complex tics include stereotyped facial gestures, hitting one's self, touching, or echolalia.

Tourette's syndrome is characterized by numerous motor and vocal tics that occur at varying frequencies and that change over time. Frequently the head is involved, along with other parts of the body, and these are almost always accompanied by vocal tics, such as barking, grunting, and coprolalia (uttering obscenities). This disorder usually appears in childhood and is apparently the result of CNS dysfunction, possibly genetic. It has been associated with obsessive compulsive disorder (Cummings & Frankel, 1985) and with learning disabilities (Lerer, 1987). This finding raises the possiblity that all three disorders are the result of similar CNS dysfunction.

Tourette's is a chronic condition with periods of exacerbation and remission. Severity of the disorder varies. As can be imagined, function in all performance spheres is impaired to a great extent in the most severe cases. However, medication (neuroleptics) in combination with education, pychological counseling, and other support can be valuable (Lerer, 1987). Chronic motor or vocal tic is much more limited, usually to a single motor or vocal tic. Severity of symptoms and of occupational impairment is much less than with Tourette's syndrome.

Transient tic disorder is most often a single tic, such as eye-blinking or another facial tic. Tics appear during childhood or adolescence but disappear within a year. Tics may be precursors to Tourette's, may disappear completely, or they may be intermittent throughout life. Tics are common among children, and many seem to resolve themselves in time (Lerer, 1987).

Elimination Disorders

This category includes functional encopresis (inability to control feces), and functional enuresis (inability to control urine). The lack of control may be voluntary or involuntary. For the diagnosis to be made, the child must be at least 4 (encopresis) or 5 (enuresis), with correlating mental age. Thus, it will not be diagnosed in retarded individuals who may lack both motor control and intelligence to be readily trained. For both disorders, the problem may be transient (e.g., caused by the stress of a new sibling or hospitalization) or may become chronic. In making this diagnosis, it is vital to rule out possible physical problems, such as urinary tract infections.

Speech Disorders not Elsewhere Classified

The two disorders included in this category are cluttering and stuttering. Cluttering is an abnormally rapid rate of speech which is difficult to comprehend. Phrasing is usually peculiar, adding to the problem. It may occur along with learning and sensory disabilities, and there may be a family history of the problem.

Stuttering is an impairment of speech fluency. This may be characterized by an inability to produce specific sounds or an inability to control repetitions of sounds or words. As the disorder becomes established, anxiety about speaking appears, exacerbating the problem. This disorder may also appear along with learning disabilities. To some extent this seems to be a genetic disorder, and stress as an etiology has been largely ruled out. Stress may, however, make stuttering worse. Depending on the severity of the stutter, performance may be minimally or severely impaired.

Stuttering has been examined extensively, and it now seems clear that a biological component is present. Some manual performance is impaired in stutterers (Webster, 1988), and articulation problems and delays in language development are common (Homzie, Lindsay, Simpson, & Hasenstab, 1988). There is also a family tendency toward stuttering (Homzie et al, 1988). Factors that do not appear related include central auditory processing (Anderson, Hood, & Sellers, 1988), and sensory perceptual and memory processing (Carpenter & Sommers, 1987).

Functional impairment depends on the severity of the stuttering, the determination of the individual, and the understanding of others. Such activities as leisure pursuits may be more difficult (Black, 1987) because of communication difficulties, but this is not automatically the case.

Other Disorders of Infancy, Childhood, and Adolescence

This category includes four disorders that do not readily fit anywhere else. They are elective mutism, identity disorder, reactive attachment disorder of infancy or early childhood, and stereotypy/habit disorder. Elective mutism is a refusal to talk in one or more situations, after it is clear that the child can speak. Although it is rare, it can be quite disabling in children in whom it occurs.

Identity disorder is reflected by an inability to form a clear sense of self. It may be demonstrated by an inability to formulate a coherent set of goals, friendships, moral values, or religious identification. Although this uncertainty is common in adolescence, it should begin to resolve itself by late adolescence. The diagnosis is typically reserved for later adolescence and early adulthood.

Disturbance of social relatedness in early childhood is characteristic of reactive attachment disorder. It is believed to be the result of severely inadequate care during infancy and early childhood and is characterized by lack of eye contact, lack of engagement in game playing, failure to attempt communication, and apathy. Poor muscle tone and weak reflexes are also present. Frequently this condition coexists with failure to thrive.

Stereotypy/habit disorder is demonstrated by repetitive nonfunctional behaviors, such as head banging. The activities are usually intentional and may cause injury to the child or interfere with activity.

Somatoform Disorders

These include body dysmorphic disorder, conversion disorder, hypochondriasis, somatization disorder, and somatoform pain disorder. These disorders are important to understand, as they frequently present in settings other than mental health facilities.

Body dysmorphic disorder reflects an obsessive dissatisfaction with a portion of the body. The individual may, for example, believe that his or her nose is ugly, face too wrinkled. There may be some minor anomaly with regard to the feature in question, but this disorder appears in normal-looking individuals. The result is often frequent visits to plastic surgeons, with dissatisfaction with surgical outcomes. Extreme functional impairment is rare, but may occur when the individual becomes so fixated on the "disfigurement" that other activities are excluded.

Conversion disorder is characterized by a loss of body function or physical impairment that suggests a physical disorder, in the absence of physical findings. The individual does not intentionally produce the physical symptom, but it will lack some features of the true physical condition. Baker and Silver (1987), in discussing hysterical paraplegia, note that accompanying sensory deficits do not fit an anatomical pattern, and that reflexes remain normal. Conversion reactions appear suddenly and often as a result of identifiable psychosocial stressors. Often the individual also has a histrionic personality disorder. In some instances there is also a lack of concern about the condition, "la belle indifference" (Nemiah, 1988). This attitude is quite striking as the individual is apparently unworried by a sudden paralysis, loss of hearing, and so on. Furthermore, sudden, rapid recovery may occur. Suggestion appears to be an effective treatment (Hafeiz, 1980).

Obsessive worry about physical condition is the defining feature of hypochondriasis. The fears are unwarranted by any physical finding, though in the absence of physical findings the individual is likely to assume the physician has not done enough. The individual makes frequent visits to the physician and to change doctors often as he or she assumes that care is inadequate or improper. This is usually a chronic condition, and impairs performance in all spheres to some extent. Those around the individual become annoyed by the obsession with physical worries, and the individual misses work because of physical concerns. In severe cases, the individual may decide to become an invalid and refuse to function for fear of "further harm" to physical condition.

An initial diagnosis of hypochondriasis may result in one of four different presentations (Idzorek, 1975): a warning of future psychiatric or physical dysfunction; a symptom of psychosis; a symptom of depression; and a "true" hypochondriasis. Obviously, making these distinctions can be difficult but vital to treatment. Hypochondriasis has been linked to depression, anxiety, and paranoid reactions (Hyer, Gouveia, Harrison, Warsaw, & Coutsouridis, 1987).

Although hypochondriasis appears to respond well to antianxiety medication (Kellner, 1983), particularly in individuals with disorder of short duration and without accompanying personality disorders, these patients can be very frustrating to care providers (Idzorek, 1975). Recognition that these are individuals who typically lack self-esteem and social skills, and need inordinate amounts of attention can help shift focus to needs and away from annoying behaviors.

Somatization disorder is characterized by multiple physical complaints over a period of years with no accompanying physical disorder. The individual seeks care for the specific disorder, presenting complaints in a vague or dramatic way. There is usually a pattern of intensive investigation of these complaints, with no positive findings. As with hypochondriacs, physician switching is common. Unlike hypochondriasis, where there is simply generalized fear that "something" may be wrong or go wrong, these individuals have specific, though unwarranted, physical complaints. The disorder is more common in women (Guze, Cloninger, Martin, & Clayton, 1986) and has been thought to parallel antisocial personality, which is much more common in men. Prognosis for Briquet's syndrome, the most common somatization disorder, is poor (Guze et al., 1986), with 80% having the same diagnosis 6 to 12 years later.

Somatoform pain disorder is the preoccupation with pain when there is no physical reason for such pain. It often occurs in individuals with a history of conversion reactions, and, like other disorders in this group, occurs in the absence of any positive physical findings. In some cases, it may develop following a physical trauma, but continues once the physical problem is resolved.

Dissociative Disorders

Multiple personality disorders, psychogenic fugue, psychogenic amnesia, and depersonalization disorder are included in this group. These disorders are striking and have frequently been portrayed in movies and television programs as "mental illness" in a global sense.

Rate of occurrence is not well-established. Some researchers believe multiple personality disorder (MPD) is quite rare, whereas others believe it is common but frequently misdiagnosed (Kluft, 1986).

A common thread in MPD is a history of child abuse (Kluft, 1986). The analytic explanation of the phenomenon is that the individual develops different personas as a defense mechanism (Kluft, 1988). For example, one personality may not remember an anxiety-provoking event that is "managed" by another, or one may express anger that is frightening to the dominant personality. Personalities tend to be separate from each other, and may be very highly developed. They seem to reflect different facets of the individual that are split or dissociated from the primary personality. This primary personality is often amnestic for the other personalities.

The goal of treatment is most often unification, i.e., reintegration of the separate personalities into one functional whole (Kluft, 1988). Hypnotherapy and cognitive therapy are among those reported effective (Ross & Gahan, 1988). Function depends on the extent and frequency with which dissociative reactions occur in the individual. Some individuals with MPD are quite functional (Kluft, 1986), whereas others are incapacitated.

Sexual Disorders

There are two main groups of sexual disorders, paraphilias and sexual dysfunctions. Paraphilias are characterized by sexual arousal in response to objects or situations that are not normally part of sexual activity, with accompanying problems relating in normal sexual activity. These include pedophilia, sexual sadism and masochism, transvestic fetishism, and others. Sexual dysfunctions represent problems in engaging in sexual relationships, including sexual aversion, inhibited orgasm, dyspareunia, premature ejaculation, and so on. Functional impairment is primarily in the area of sexual relationships, but may extend to heterosexual relationships more generally if the sexual problem begins to generalize to feelings of low self-esteem or anxiety.

Sleep Disorders

Sleep disorders will not be diagnosed in situations where the duration of the problem is brief. Many individuals have periods of sleep disturbance when stressed or ill, but for most people these are brief and transient. In some cases, though, the problem persists, either in the form of dysomnia (difficulty sleeping) or hypersomnia (excessive sleeping). The *DSM-III-R* listing does not include physical disorders, such as narcolepsy, but only those which are thought to be psychogenic.

Also included in this category are sleep-wake disturbances, in which the normal diurnal cycle of sleep is disturbed, and parasomnias, which are characterized by abnormal events during sleep, e.g., nightmares and sleep-walking. Again, the problem must be of several months duration for a diagnosis to be made, as occasional problems are not unusual.

Factitious Disorders

These are physical or psychological disorders that are intentionally produced and under the voluntary control of the individual. The concept of voluntary control is somewhat problematic here, however. Although individuals may actively induce a symptom (through ingestion of drugs, for example), they are not able to control the impulse to do so. This group does not include malingering, in which the individual both produces the symptom voluntarily and wishes to do so at a conscious level. The best known factitious disorder is Munchausen syndrome. This syndrome is characterized by numerous hospitalizations for a variety of symptoms, with accompanying physical signs, such as nausea and vomiting, rashes, bleeding, all of which have been induced by the individual. Symptoms are dramatic but vague, and individuals have extensive knowledge of hospital routines. They are difficult to manage once hospitalized, because they are both noncompliant and demanding. It appears that these individuals are socially isolated and derive most of their social satisfaction by being taken care of in an inpatient setting. When confronted with the real nature of their symptoms, they may leave against medical advice, often to seek readmittance elsewhere.

There is much to suggest that these disorders may be prodromal to psychosis, particularly when the disorder feigned is a psychosis (Hay, 1983; Pope, Jonas, & Jones, 1982). Long term outcomes are poor, particularly since many of these individuals have accompanying personality disorders.

Impulse Control Disorders
Not Elsewhere Classified

These include intermittent explosive disorder, kleptomania, pathological gambling, pyromania, and trichotillomania. In each, the individual is driven to engage in a behavior that is damaging to self or others, which he or she is unable to control. Origin of the disorders is not well understood, but interference with function is common. Explosive disorder, kleptomania, and pyromania may ultimately result in imprisonment, whereas pathological gambling is damaging to social and work relationships. Trichotillomania (pulling out one's own hair) is the least damaging of these disorders, although it may indicate poor self-esteem which is reflected in other performance.

Adjustment Disorders

These disorders may appear at any time in life and can be directly linked to a stressful event. By definition, function is impaired as the individual has difficulty with social, vocational, school, or leisure activities. Stressors include such things as divorce, loss of a job, physical illness, or natural disaster. The severity of the disorder is not necessarily in proportion to the severity of the stressor but rather a reflection of the individual's ability to cope. Anxiety, depression, conduct disorder, and physical complaints may accompany the disorder. These symptoms are self-limiting, occuring within 3 months of the stressor, with a duration of no more than 6 months prior to seeking conduct disorder, outcome is worse (Andreasen & Hoenk, 1982).

Studies of the validity of the category provide evidence of face, descriptive, and predictive validity among adults (Andreasen & Hoenk, 1982). It is clear, for example, that the majority of adults improve in the absence of continued stress. It is less clear that this is a valid diagnostic category for adolescents.

Codes for Conditions not Attributable to a Mental Disorder that are a Focus of Attention or Treatment

There are times when individuals enter treatment for specific problems that are not directly tied to psychiatric disorders. Academic or marital problems, uncomplicated bereavement, occupational (vocational) problems, and parent-child problems are among those on this list. Although individuals seeking treatment for these problems may have accompanying disorders, the difficulty may not have resulted from the mental disorder. As an example, an individual who has had anxiety problems may still experience uncomplicated bereavement as a result of loss of a spouse.

Implications for Occupational Therapy

For each of these disorders occupational therapy may be warranted if the disorder impacts negatively on function, the disorder impacts negatively on self-esteem, or remediation requires learning a new set of performance skills.

As an example, transsexual individuals may have performed quite adequately in both work and social spheres, but have suffered severe difficulty in terms of self-esteem and self-concept. Should they opt for sex reassignment, a whole set of new skills will be needed. The well-publicized case of Renee Richards is an example. She was a successful male physician, married with several children. This was an extremely uncomfortable role, however, and she ultimately chose sex reassignment. This necessitated, among many other concerns, considerable education about how to behave as a female.

A more commonly encountered example would be individuals with hypochondriasis. Function is typically impaired as the individual worries about health and takes to bed with every real or imagined ailment. Self-esteem is likely to be impaired, either as a precursor to the disorder or as a consequence of the inability to function and the inevitable annoyance of others. These individuals clearly need a new set of behaviors that can provide a source of satisfaction and improved self-esteem. In the absence of such learning, remediation of symptoms is difficult. This is because hypochondriasis is so often a plea for attention from individuals who have very low self-regard.

Review of disorders in this chapter provides an opportunity to restate the occupational therapy view of dysfunction. This view cuts across lines drawn by medical diagnosis. Issues of self-esteem, self-concept, and performance appear almost regardless of diagnosis. Although the degree of impairment and the specific nature of the impairment differ, these themes are consistent and primary to the occupational therapist.

References

Andreasen, N.C. & Hoenk, P.R. (1982). The predictive value of adjustment disorders: A follow-up study. *American Journal of Psychiatry, 139,* 584-590.

Anderson, J.M., Hoods, S.B., & Sellers, D.E. (1988). Central Auditory Processing abilities of adolescent and preadolescent stuttering and nonstuttering children. *Journal of Fluency Disorders, 13,* 199-214.

Baker & Silver, J.R. (1987). Hysterical paraplegia. *Journal of Neurology, Neurosurgery, and Psychiatry, 50,* 375-382.

Black, J.A. (1987). A comparative study of the perception of freedom-in-leisure between stuttering and nonstuttering individuals. *Journal of Fluency Disorders, 12,* 239-248.

Carpenter, M. & Sommers, R.K. (1987). Unisensory and bisensory perceptual and memory processing in stuttering adults and normal speakers. *Journal of Fluency Disorders, 12,* 291-304.

Cummings, J.L. & Frankel, M. (1985). Gilles de la Tourette syndrome and the neurological basis of obsessions and compulsions. *Biological Psychiatry, 20,* 1117-1126.

Edelman, R.J. (1986). Adaptive training for existing male transsexual gender role: A case history. *Journal of Sex Research, 22,* 514-531.

Guze, S.B., Cloninger, C.R., Martin, R.L., & Clayton, P.J. (1986). A follow-up and family study of Briquet's syndrome. *British Journal of Psychiatry, 149,* 17-23.

Hafeiz, H.B. (1980). Hysterical conversion: A prognostic study. *British Journal of Psychiatry, 136,* 548-551.

Hay, G.G. (1983). Feigned psychosis—A review of the simulation of mental illness. *British Journal of Psychiatry, 143,* 8-10.

Homzie, M.J., Lindsay, J.S., Simpson, J., & Hasenstab, S. (1988). Concomitant speech, language, and learning problems in adult stutterers and in members of their families. *Journal of Fluency Disorders, 13,* 261-277.

Hyer, L., Gouveia, I., Harrison, W.R., Warsa, J., & Coutsouridis, D. (1987). Depression, anxiety, paranoid reactions, hypochondriasis, and cognitive decline of later-life inpatients. Journal of Gerontology, 42, 92-94.

Idzorek, S. (1975). A functional classification of hypochondriasis with specific recommendations for treatment. *Southern Medical Journal, 68,* 1326-1332.

Kellner, R. (1983). Prognosis of treated hypochondriasis: A clinical study. *Acta Psychiatrica Scandinavia, 67,* 69-79.

Khanna, S., Desai, N.G., & Channabasavanna, S.M. (1987). Case study: A treatment package for transsexualism. *Behavior Therapy, 2,* 193-199.

Kluft, R.P. (1988). The postunification treatment of multiple personality disorder: First findings. *American Journal of Psychotherapy, 42,* 212-227.

Kluft, R.P. (1986). High-functioning multiple personality patients: Three cases. *The Journal of Nervous and Mental Disease, 174.*

Kockott, G. & Fahrner, E.M. (1987). Transsexuals who have not undergone surgery: A follow-up study. *Archives of Sexual Behavior, 16,* 511-522.

Lerer, R.J. (1987). Motor tics, Tourette syndrome, and learning disabilities. *Journal of Learning Disabilities, 20,* 266-267.

Nemiah, J.C. (1988). Psychoneurotic disorders. In A.M. Nicholi (Ed.), *The New Harvard Guide to Psychiatry.* Cambridge, MA: Belknap Press, pp. 234-258.

Pope, H.G., Jonas, J.M., & Jones, B. (1982). Factitious psychosis: Phenomenology, family history, and long-term outcome of nine patients. *American Journal of Psychiatry, 139,* 1480-1483.

Ross, C.A. & Gahan, P. (1988). Cognitive analysis of multiple personality disorder. *American Journal of Psychotherapy, 42,* 229-239.

Webster, W.G. (1988). Neural mechanisms underlying stuttering: Evidence from bimanual handwriting performance. *Brain and Language, 33,* 226-244.

Chapter 11
Psychotropic Medications
Phillip James Fischer, MD

Introduction

One cornerstone of patient care is the skillful and enlightened use of psychotropic medication. The purpose of this chapter is to introduce the reader to some general principles about psychotropic medications: indications and contraindications, advantages and disadvantages, effects and side effects. This information is important to the members of the multidisciplinary team to enable them to reinforce gains, recognize side effects, and communicate any perceived impediment to maximal functioning of the patient to the treatment team.

This chapter will be divided into several sections. There will be a brief overview of the early development of psychopharmacology and a discussion of the use of the laboratory results to guide decisions about medication. There will be a section for each of the major psychoactive drug classes with the primary focus being on the general adult population. Issues around the use of these agents in children and elders will be touched on briefly. Finally, general principles that affect decisions about use of pychotropic medications will be discussed.

History

Mankind has been searching for ways to reduce the pain and suffering of psychic distress throughout history. Each culture has had its armamentarium of treatments. Ancient peoples bored holes in the skull to let out evil spirits (trephination). The use of alcohol to reduce dysphoria, herbal remedies, opiates, cocaine, marijuana, coffee, tobacco, and many other plant derived psychotropic agents have been used as folk remedies. The effects of some of these compounds have been studied and many have found their way into traditional medicine.

The chance discoveries of the anti-manic effect of lithium and of chlorpromazine's (Thorazine) antipsychotic properties signaled the beginning of modern psychopharmacology. In the ensuing 40 years many new drugs have been developed that have improved the quality of life in patients afflicted with a variety of psychiatric disorders. The discovery and development of these compounds started with unexpected clinical findings of efficacy. Ongoing research has improved understanding of basic psychopharmacology and drug side effects, leading to the ongoing development of better drugs and suggesting biologic theories of causation for some psychiatric illnesses.

Chlorpromazine (Thorazine) was synthesized as an antihistamine in 1952 and was found to produce an easily arousable sedation that was useful as a preanesthetic (Davis, 1985). The observation that it produced behavioral changes led to experimental trials of the drug in psychotic patients. Many of these "hopeless cases" experienced dramatic improvement. Since that time the further development of newer antipsychotic drugs has permitted many individuals to function outside of psychiatric hospitals instead of being institutionalized for life.

Both major classes of antidepressants, tricyclics and monoamine oxidase inhibitors (MAOI), were discovered accidentally. Imipramine (Tofranil), the first of the tricyclic antidepressants, was discovered while researchers were looking for a better chlorpromazine-like drug (Davis, 1985). It was found that though imipramine was ineffective in schizophrenics, it did produce improvement in depressed patients. The first MAOI, ipronozid, was used to treat tuberculosis and was observed to produce an elevated mood in tuberculosis patients (Davis, 1985).

Many of the psychotropic drugs were discovered by chance when they were given to see what would happen, or were given for one condition and were observed to be helpful in a different disorder. Cade, an Australian state hospital superintendent, in 1949 tried lithium experimentally and found that it reduced mania. The history of the development of antidepressant and antipsychotic drugs points up the fact that major scientific discoveries can evolve as consequences of clinical investigation rather than deductions from animal models (Davis, 1985).

Role of Laboratory Testing in Diagnosis and Medication Use

Regardless of the type of medication, practitioners are increasingly better able to make decisions because of expanding knowledge about drug actions. When psychotropic medications were first discovered, they were used largely on a trial and error basis. Now, however, laboratory tests are routinely being used to rule in or out other medical conditions that can mimic or complicate psychiatric illnesses. Increasingly, the laboratory results are used to aid in diagnosis and to monitor the safety and efficacy of drug treatment. For example, the dexamethasone suppression test, a test that measures plasma cortisone levels, when correlated with clinical findings, can help diagnose major depression, and as test results revert to "normal" the clinician can judge if the proper treatment was selected. The ability to monitor blood levels of psychotropic drugs can help the clinician know if the proper dosage is being prescribed to get the patient to a therapeutic level.

This has taken some of the guesswork out of prescribing. In the past, a psychiatrist might select an antidepressant, for example, and adjust the dose based on clinical response, side effects, and published data on the acceptable dosage range. This sometimes led to improper dosing and subsequent treatment failure.

For example, under earlier guidelines the dosage range for the antidepressant imipramine (Tofranil) was considered to be between 50 mg to 350 mg per day. It was thought that below 50 mg per day there would be no response and more than 350 mg per day was thought to be toxic and unlikely to yield further significant improvement. The former practice was to start the drug out at a low dose and increase it every few days until one of three outcomes was observed, namely:

1. A clear clinical improvement was noted, in which case the drug would be maintained at this level for 3 to 9 months;
2. Intolerable side effects occurred, in which case the drug would be discontinued and another drug tried; or
3. The dose was increased to what was believed to be the maximum allowed. If there was no improvement in 4 to 6 weeks, another drug was tried. Sometimes, what might have been considered treatment resistant depression was really under treatment.

Now it is possible to tailor treatment with more precision. It is now known that therapeutic blood levels can be seen at what was previously thought to be extremely low doses, 25 mg to 50 mg of imipramine, with good clinical improvement. In principle, it is always best to use the lowest effective dose possible, especially in children, the elderly, and persons with medical illnesses. Conversely, the clinician now has the flexibility of exceeding the upper limits of dosage, turning many "failed drug trials" into positive outcomes and in shorter time.

The laboratory can also be used to detect medication noncompliance, drug abuse, and to monitor blood levels for relapse prevention. In addition to blood and urine parameters, there are several other diagnostic tools available to the clinician today, including EEG and polysomnography, computerized axial tomography (CAT scan), magnetic resonance imaging (MRI), position emission tomography (PET scan), topical brain mapping, and psychological tests (psychometrics) (Gold, Potash, & Extein, 1984).

The laboratory, then, is an increasingly vital part of modern psychiatric treatment and as refinements and new technology develop, will be even more important.

The psychotropic drugs to be discussed in this chapter have proven efficacy as well as the potential to cause serious adverse effects. When prescribing any medication, a careful judgment has to be based on consideration of the risk versus benefit ratio.

Specific Drug Classifications

Antidepressants

Pathophysiology of Depressive illness

Before discussing specific agents, it is important to have an overview of what is believed about "biological" depression. As a diagnosis, depression implies an underlying chemical imbalance of the central nervous system. The most commonly accepted hypothesis today is that a functional deficiency of two neurotransmitters (noreinephrine and serotonin) is important in depressive illness. These two substances, also called monamines, are contained in vesicles and stored in the presynaptic neuron (Fig. 11-1a). These monamines are discharged into the interneuronal space (synaptic cleft) and become carriers of impulse transmission to the postsynaptic neuron (Fig. 11-1b) (Hackett & Cassem, 1978). Transmission occurs when these monamines bind to the postsynaptic neuron. The binding is brief and the molecule is released back into the synaptic cleft to be reabsorbed or metabolized (Fig. 11-1c). For norepinephrine, about 50% of that stored comes from reuptake. Destruction of the unstored monoamine occurs within the cell by the monoamine oxidase enzymes and in the extracellular space by the enzymes called -methyl-transferases (Hackett & Cassem, 1978).

The complexity of the electrochemical processes necessary for normal brain function makes the possibility of dysfunction readily understandable. Failure to terminate the action of a released neurotransmitter would be likely to prolong, inhibit, or exaggerate its action. Likewise, the production and release of excess monamines or excessive sensitivity of the receptor site to the action of these neurotransmitters would produce an exaggerated effect at the cellular level, which may be seen as a clinical abnormality. On the other hand, deficient synthesis or release of neurotransmitter molecules, or decreased sensitivity of the receptor site, also would likely produce a physiologic

Figure 11-1a   Figure 11-1b   Figure 11-1c

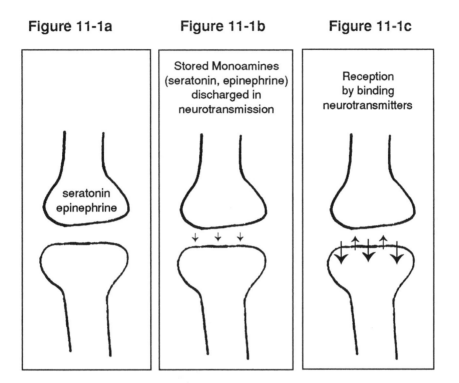

abnormality that again could be manifested clinically in abnormalities of thought processes, mood, or behavior (Hackett & Cassem, 1978). The antidepressant drugs work at the level of neurotransmission to "normalize" transmission of impulses.

Tricyclic Antidepressants

The tricyclic antidepressant drugs (TCA) such as amitriptyline (Elavil), imipramine (Tofranil), and doxepin (Sinequan, Adapin) form the mainstay of the pharmacologic treatment of depression. There are a variety of tricyclic drugs that are more or less equally effective in the treatment of depression (Table 11-1). These compounds probably work by blocking neuronal reuptake of norepinephrine and serotonin. The TCAs mainly differ in the extent and severity of their side effects. To varying degrees, all available tricyclic antidepressants block acetylcholine and consequently inhibit the parasympathetic nervous system. This cholinergic blockade by TCAs is responsible for commonly reported side effects which include blurred vision, dry mouth, reduced sweating, constipation, urinary retention, and tachycardia (Bassuk & Schoonover, 1977). Patients with cardiac diseases or other medical problems that would make them particularly vulnerable to anticholinergic drugs should be treated cautiously with TCAs. [For such patients it would be preferable to use doxepin (Sinequan) or desipramine (Norpramin) because of their lower anticholinergic potency (Roose & Glassman, 1989].

Table 11-1
Summary of Antidepressant Drugs Currently Used in the United States

Name			Avail. Preps (mgs) Oral		Comments, Advantages/ Disadvantages
Class	Generic	Trade	Tablet	Capsule	
Tricyclic Type Norepinephrine (NE) Seratonin (SHT) Inhibitors	Imipramine	Tofranil SK-Pramine Imavate Janamine	10, 25, 30	75, 100, 125, 150	
	Amitriptyline	Elavil Endep	10, 25, 50 75, 100, 150		
	Doxepin	Sinequan Adapin		10, 25, 50, 75, 100, 150	
	Amoxapine	Asendin	25, 50, 100, 150		
	Trazadone	Desyrel	50, 100, 150		
	Trimipramine	Surmontil		25, 50, 100	
	Chlorimipra- mine	Anafranil	25, 50		Not Yet Available Imipramine- like anti- obsessive
Norepinephrine (NE) Uptake In- hibitors	Desipramine	Norpramin Pertofrane	10, 25, 50, 75, 100, 150	25, 50	Metabolite of Imipramine Less sedative Frequently used as research standard
	Nortriptyline	Aventyl Pamelor		10, 25, 75	Amitriptyline Metabolite Less sedative Less hypoten- sion May have ad- vantage in el- derly

Table 11-1 *continued*
Summary of Antidepressant Drugs Currently Used in the United States

Name			Dose Range	Comments, Advantages, Disadvantages
Class	Generic	Trade		
Tricyclic Type				
NE Uptake Inhibitors	Protriptyline	Vivactil	5, 10 mg	
	Mapratoline	Ludiomil	20, 50, 75 mg	
Norepinephrine Synthesis Enhancer	Miansedin			An experimental tetracyclic not yet available in the U.S.
Norepinephrine Potentiator	Bupropion	Wellbutrin	100 mg	
				Reported advangates are: • No NE or SHT reuptake block • Non-sedative • No weight gain • Non-stimulant • Not cardiotoxic • Minimal anti- cholinergic effects • Overdose safe
	Alprazolan	Xanax	25, .5, 1 mg	Developed as an anti-anxiety drug. Few side effects. Addiction potential with prolonged use.
Norepinephrine (NE) Uptake Inhibitors				
Serotonin Uptake Inhibitors	Fluoxetine	Prozac	20 mg	Unique structure No anticholinergic efect
Monoamine Oxidase Inhibitors	Phenelzine	Nardil	15 mg	Good in resistant atypical depression. Avoid tyramine.
	Tramycypromine	Parnate	10 mg	Stimulant Avoid Tyramine

Sedation is probably the most common side effect associated with TCAs. This effect may be inconvenient or unpleasant in that it may interfere with the life functions of the patient during the day. However, this sedative side effect can be beneficial since insomnia and anxiety are frequently among the most troublesome symptoms of depression. Usually the sedation lessens over a 2 to 4 week period as the patient "adjusts" to the medication. Interestingly, this same 2 to 4 week period is when the properly dosed patient notices a subjective sense of improvement.

It should be kept in mind that TCAs may interact with a variety of other medications. The sedative effect of TCAs may be increased when they are used with a variety of CNS depressant drugs. Alcohol should be avoided since its effects will be increased and because alcohol, a CNS depressant, can worsen depression itself. Patients should be cautioned about driving or working around hazardous machinery until a functional assessment can be made (Smiley, 1987). The selection of the least sedative TCA is prudent in the patient who must be alert during the day. Frequently, giving the medication as a single evening dose can minimize this problem. Although the sedative effect is usually transient, a trial of a different class of drug may be needed to identify the drug with the least sedative side effects. TCAs interfere with the antihypertensive effect of several types of blood pressure medications, specifically guanethidine and clonodine (Bassuk & Schoonover, 1977). If a TCA is indicated, the antihypertensive drug can be changed in cooperation with the patient's primary care specialist.

TCAs can produce orthostatic (postural) hypotension, (the transient and precipitous lowering of blood pressure as the patient arises from a supine to standing position). This can lead to blackouts, which can further lead to falls and serious injury (Smiley, 1987). The elderly are particularly prone to this side effect, which can lead to devastating injuries, particularly fractured hips and wrists. Therefore, it is extremely important to discuss this and the other side effects carefully with the patient and, if possible, with a significant family member or friend.

The anticholinergic effects of tricyclic drugs can be additive with anticholinergic effects of other agents that medical patient may be receiving, eg, antiparkisonian drugs. TCAs can also produce or worsen cardiac arrhythmias. Therefore, it is a good idea to obtain baseline and follow up EKGs, especially in the elderly (Roose & Glassman, 1989).

Some patients receiving tricyclic antidepressants may become confused or agitated. This effect is linked either to their anticholinergic effect or to the ability of these drugs to uncover a previously unrecognized psychotic disturbance. Larger doses of tricyclic drugs may cause toxic psychosis with auditory and visual hallucinations (Davis, 1985). Visual hallucinations are assumed to be organically based until proven otherwise so drugs must be considered as a possible cause. Some patients with an unrecognized underlying bipolar disorder may experience a "manic switch" or acute manic psychosis after treatment for depressive illness with tricyclic drugs (Davis, 1985). Occasional confusion and less well-defined memory deficits have been associated with tyicyclic antidepressants. Table 11-2 summarizes side effects.

Table 11-2
Summary of Antidepressant Side Effects

Dry Mouth Palpitations Tachycardia Heart Block Myocardial Infarction	Vomiting Constipation Sedation Agitation	Aggravation of Narrow Angle Glaucoma Urinary Retention Paralytic ileus

Loss of accomodation
  (blurred vision)
Orthostatic hypoten-
  sion
Fainting
Nausea
	Hallucinations, delu-
	  sions in latent psy-
	  chosis
	Diarrhea
	Black tongue
	Edema
		Peculiar Taste
		Skin rash
		Galactorrhea
		Gynecomastria
		Bone marrow depres-
		  sion

The antidepressant drugs do not markedly influence the normal organism in a baseline state but rather correct an abnormal condition. The action may be similar to aspirin, which will lower a fever but does not lower normal temperatures (Davis, 1985). The TCAs and MAOIs are antidepressants, not general euphoriants or stimulants. Thus, although imipramine has marked antidepressant action on depressed psychiatric patients, good evidence indicates that it has little euphoriant action on normal persons (Hackett & Cassem, 1978). It is known that when the MAIOs are used to treat high blood pressure, most patients do not experience marked mental effects. In contrast, amphetamine is a euphoriant and a stimulant, but is not an antidepressant in the precise sense of the word (Hackett & Cassem, 1978).

The TCAs - imipramine (Tofranil), amitriptyline (Elavil), desipramine (Norpramin), nortriptyline (Pamelor), protriptyline (Vivactil) - are structurally similar to the phenothiazines. That similarity emphasizes the importance of minor structural differences in drugs in the production of critical changes in pharmacological activity. The great majority of the TCAs block the reuptake of norepinephrine (NE) or serotonin (5-hydroxytryptomine, 5HT), down-regulate GLB-NE receptors, and produce the same range of effects. The pharmacology of the tricyclic-type is complex because those drugs also affect histamine-2 receptors (Kalinowsky, Hippius, & Helmfried, 1982). As a result of these properties there is a compensatory decrease of NE synthesis, presumably as a result of noradrenergic potentiation.

The TCAs are readily absorbed from the gastrointestinal tract. In humans, imipramine (Tofranil), amitriptyline (Elavil), chlorimipramine (Anafranil), and doxepin (Sinequan, Adapin), are partially metabolized to their respective desmethyl derivation. These metabolites are therapeutically active and have fewer side effects (Davis, 1985).

Clinical Effects

In normal persons, tricyclic drugs produce slight sedation; however, in severely depressed psychotic patients they produce a striking improvement in behavior and marked lessening of depression, often 3 to 10 days after the start of treatment. Using the drug doubles the chance of recovery after 3 to 4 weeks of treatment. Patients who do not respond after receiving an adequate dose of the drug for 3 weeks probably will not respond at all. Furthermore, the degree of response in the first week predicts the ultimate therapeutic response (Bassuk & Schoonover, 1977).

Monoamine Oxidase Inhibitors

This group of psychoactive agents is frequently effective in the treatment of severe endogenous depression, panic disorders, and in the atypical depression associated with borderline personality disorder (Par, 1987). These agents are divided into two categories: hydrazines and non-hydrazines. The hydrazines include isocarboxazid and phenlzine (Nardil). The only nonhydrazine in use is tranylcypromine (Parnate). The structural difference is clinically important. Tranylcypromine has somewhat stimulant amphetamine-like qualities that often produce clinical improvement in about 10 days. Tranylcypromine, however, has a greater degree of side effects, particularly of the cardiovascular system. The hydrazines are effective within 3 to 4 weeks and have a lower incidence of side effects (Bassuk & Schoonover, 1977).

The MAOIs inhibit many enzyme systems. They elevate body levels of epinephrine, norepinephrine, 5HT, and dopamine by irreversibly binding to the degradation enzymes of these substances. This process greatly increases the body's available biogenic amines. It is hypothesized that this CNS effect is responsible for the antidepressant activity. The MAOIs can produce many serious side effects and should be prescribed only by experienced practitioners (Bassuk & Schoonover, 1977).

Cardiovascular side effects of the MAOIs, including orthostatic hypotension, tachycardia, and palpitations, can be life-threatening. In cardiac patients, these agents can eliminate or delay the onset of angina pectoris by blocking the response of the cardiovascular system to exercise (Jefferson, 1989). This effect can promote conditions that predispose to myocardial infarction (Jefferson, 1989). The most worrisome cardiovascular side effect is hypertension. This can occur at therapeutic doses, but usually occurs when high doses of the MAOIs are taken, when the drug is combined with a tricyclic antidepressant or sympathomimetic agents (such as cough and cold preparations), or when tyramine (found in a variety of foods) is consumed. The hypertension is caused by the release of catecholamines in the peripheral nervous system. A severe, atypical headache is usually the first sign and may foretell an impending hypertensive crisis that can lead to a cerebrovascular accident (stroke) and death.

Eating foods with a high tyramine content is a major concern. Tyramine is a fermentation by-product, so foods with aged protein should be avoided. Aged cheeses, meats, and fish, most alcoholic beverages, especially beer and red wine, and overripe fruits and vegetables should be avoided. Consumption of chocolate and coffee should be limited.

MAOIs and many pharmacologic agents are synergistic and can result in hypertensive crisis. These include amphetamines, ephedrine, procaine preparations, such as Novacain, epinephrine, methyldopa, meperidine (Demerol), and phenylpropanolamine, which is found in many over-the-counter cold preparations. Patients must be informed to check with their psychiatrist before taking any other medication while on MAOIs. An instruction sheet is usually provided to the patient as part of the informed consent. Tricyclic antidepressants should be discontinued at least 7 days before a trial of MAOIs and vice versa. Fluoxetine (Prozac) should be discontinued 5 to 6 weeks before starting MAOI. MAOI and TCA are occasionally combined for severe, treatment-resistant depressions under special and controlled circumstances. Fortunately, hypertensive reaction is very rare and can be reversed with prompt administration of an antidote, phentolamine.

The precipitation of hypomania or mania can occur. The overall side effect profile is similar to the TCAs and is summarized in Table 11-1.

Overall, the MAOIs are safe and effective in experienced hands, with proper precautions, and in patients able and willing to comply with restrictions.

Newer Antidepressants

Fluoxetine (Prozac) represents the first of a new class of antidepressants that selectively inhibits neuronal uptake of serotonin. Recent literature suggests that serotonin may be the most important neurotransmitter implicated in depression. Prozac has now been used in the United States for a year and is becoming one of the most prescribed antidepressants because of its relative safety (Cooper, 1988), favorable side to effect profile, and patient acceptance. In addition to its antidepressant effects, this agent has shown promising results in the treatment of obsessive-compulsive disorder and bulimia.

Prozac has very little anticholinergic activity, therefore there is a low incidence of drowsiness, dry mouth, cognitive impairment, constipation, or weight gain. The most common side effects are transient nausea, nervousness, and insomnia. In comparison studies, Prozac is as effective as the TCAs (Schuckit, 1988).

Buproprion (Wellbutrin) is an antidepressant of the animodetone class and is chemically unrelated to other known antidepressant agents. The exact neurochemical mechanism of the antidepressant effect is unknown. It exerts minimal receptor blockage, i.e., it does not block reception of impulses of the synapse. Buproprion's efficacy is equal to the the TCAs, with most patients responding in 3 weeks. The adverse effects most frequently observed are agitation, dry mouth, insomnia, nausea, constipation, and tremor. In 1985, this drug was voluntarily withdrawn from the US market because of concern about the potential for seizures. Subsequent studies have shown this to be a safe drug but it is not recommended for use in anyone with a seizure potential nor in those with a history of bulimia or anorexia nervosa (Mahta, 1983).

Antianxiety Agents

Anxiety is a universal response to stress and is necessary for effective functioning and coping. It is experienced as a state of tension accompanied by feelings of dread and potential danger. However, in some individuals the symptom complex is so severe that the patient is immobilized and dysfunctional. The decision whether to medicate anxiety is complex, and clearly, medication is one modality that usually should be integrated into a more comprehensive plan. Antianxiety drugs produce symptomatic relief of anxiety. Even if the anxiety is adaptive, an antianxiety agent may improve the patient's ability to cope, or enhance the effectiveness of other types of treatment. Antianxiety drugs are useful in only a few situations and always in the context of an ongoing relationship between the patient, the prescribing physician, and the interdisciplinary treatment team. Generally, they should be used for short term administration. Major types of antianxiety agents are listed in Table 11-3.

Table 11-3
Antianxiety Drugs

Class	Chemical Name	Trade Name	Dosage
Benzodiazepine	Chlordiazepoxide	Librium	10-100mg/d
	Diazepam	Valium	2-40mg/d
	Oxazepam	Serax	15-90mg/d
	Flurazepam	Dalmane	15-30mgd
	Alprazolam	Xanax	.1254mg/d
	Clorazepate	Tranzene	15-60mg/d
Antihistamines	Cyclizine	Maverzine	
	Hydroxyzine	Atarax, Visteril	75-400mg/d
	Diphenhydramine	Benedryl	25-100mg/d
Barbituates		Amytal	
		Seconal	
		Nembutal	
Carbamate	Meprobamate		400mg

Benzodiazepines

The benzodiazepines have been the most prescribed of all psychotropic drugs for the past 20 years. The currently marketed benzodiazepine are listed in Table 11-3. In 1985, 6 of the 25 most prescribed drugs were benzodiazepines (Sussman & Chou, 1988). In that year, benzodiazepines accounted for one in every two prescriptions among adults. Such extensive use of benzodiazepines is associated with considerable controversy. Critics of benzodiazepines cite two properties of the drugs that make them susceptible to abuse, i.e., they produce euphoriant effects and have a rapid onset of action. Others argue that abuse and habituation is relatively infrequent and limited primarily to those with histories of substance abuse (Shader & Greenblatt, 1984). The negative publicity surrounding the benzodiazepines has produced a number of problems, foremost among them a hesitancy to prescribe the medications in cases where their benefits clearly outweigh their potential harm. Sensationalized accounts of diazepam (Valium) abuse have served to deflect attention from the therapeutically useful role benzodiazepines can play (Sussman & Chou, 1988). They have also obscured awareness of some important liabilities associated with the class as a whole, some of which are more prevalent and clinically significant than abuse per se.

Table 11-4
Therapeutic Effects of Benzodiazepines

• Anxiety Reduction	• Anesthesia
• Sedation	• Amnesia
• Anticonvulsant Activity	• Antipanic Activity
• Muscle Relaxation	• Antidepressant
• Antistress Effect	• Alcohol Withdrawal

Table 11-5
Side Effects of Benzodiazepines

• Sedation	• Impaired Concentration
• Psychomotor	• Weakness
• Impairment	• Impaired sexual function
• Depression	• Amnesia
• Amnesia	• Agitation (rare)
• Dependence	

The widespread use of benzodiazepines derives from their therapeutic usefulness for a broad range of indications (Table 11-4). Most reviews emphasize their effectiveness as antianxiety agents. Specific effects include reduction in worry, shakiness, physiologic symptoms, and panic attacks (Sussman & Chou, 1988). They appear to be more effective in people suffering from severe anxiety and appear to have little impact on those with low anxiety levels. There is conflicting evidence about the efficacy of long term benzodiazepine therapy. Some studies do not demonstrate continued effects beyond 6 months, although others suggest some anxious patients benefit from life-long treatment (Haskell, Cole, & Schniebolk, 1986).

The inability to dissociate the sedative from the anxiolytic effects of benzodiazepines leaves unanswered the degree to which these drugs specifically reduce anxiety, rather than reducing overall central nervous system arousal. Some evidence suggests that the initial effects of benzodiazepines are sedative with anxiolytic action appearing after about a week of treatment.

Tolerance to the sedative effect appears at about this time (File & Pellow, 1987).

Panic attacks have long been known to respond to treatments with antidepressants and beta-blockers, but not to treatment with standard benzodiazepines (File & Pellow, 1987). However, recent experience has shown that alprazolam (Xanax) produces significant improvement in panic disorder. Full therapeutic effects are generally achieved within the first week of treatment. Another benzodiazepine, clonazepam (Klonopin), normally used as an anticonvulsant, has been found to be an effective antipanic drug (Tesar & Rosenbaum, 1986).

Benzodiazepines also produce an anti-stress effect, blocking stress induced increases in corticosteroid concentration and plasma catecholamines (Sussman & Chou, 1988). Therefore, these drugs are often used for patients with medical disorders. Especially in coronary heart disease, the administration of antianxiety drugs may reduce the incidence of subsequent myocardial infarction.

Benzodiazepines are widely employed to help ease alcoholic withdrawal syndrome. Since these agents attach to the same receptor sites in the brain as alcohol, these agents can be substituted and then tapered off over a 5 to 7 day period.

All of the benzodiazepines produce similar pharmacologic effects. The differences among the drugs involve pharmacokinetics, such as rates of absorption, elimination half-life, pathways of metabolism and lipid solubility, factors that contribute to the overall effect by influencing the onset and duration of action. The single most important difference is elimination half-life (Sussman & Chou, 1988). Slowly eliminated drugs accumulate and lead to an increased risk of accidents and cognitive impairment. Problems of accumulation are even more problematic in the elderly because of slowed metabolic activity of the liver and kidneys, which is part of the normal aging progress. Short half-life drugs also have special risks such as a more intense withdrawal syndrome, as well as interdose rebound anxiety.

Although comparatively safe, benzodiazepines can produce a wide array of adverse effects. Psychomotor impairment may be the most lethal of all benzodiazepine related side effects. Impairment of driving skills puts drivers at nearly five times more risk of involvement in a serious accident than those not taking benzodiazepines (Linnoila, Erwin, & Brende, 1983). Global cognitive impairment in the elderly is a significant problem with long half-life anxiolytics and hypnotics accounting for the greatest incidence. The onset of impairment is often insidious, with signs of cognitive impairment becoming evident after years of treatment. Thinking ability improves once the drug is discontinued (Fang, Hinrich, & Ghonheim, 1987).

Although benzodiazepine-induced amnesia is an unwanted effect when these agents are used an anxiolytics, it is a necessary property in anesthesia as it helps the patient forget the more traumatic aspects of diagnostic and surgical procedures (O'Boyle, Barry, Fox, et al, 1982).

Other side effects include treatment-emergent depression and paradoxical aggression or mania (Lydiard, Larai, Ballenger, et al, 1987). Benzodiazepines can cause ventilatory impairment and thus should be used with extreme caution in patients with chronic obstructive lung disease.

About 40% of those who use benzodiazepines for 6 months or more show definite withdrawal on discontinuation. Some may develop dependence after only 6 weeks. Nevertheless, many patients who have been taking benzodiazepines for years do not experience withdrawal symptoms (Busto, Sellers, Naranjo, et al, 1986).

Some commonly reported withdrawal symptoms are anxiety and insomnia. Withdrawal symptoms also include tinnitus (ringing in the ears), involuntary movements, perceptual changes (increased sensitivity to environmental stimuli), confusion, and depersonalization (Busto et al, 1986).

Abrupt discontinuation of high dose therapy with diazepam produces the most severe withdrawal syndrome with disorientation, delirium, seizures, and psychotic reactions. General strategies for minimizing the clinical impact of withdrawal include stopping the drug as soon as the reason for taking it has ceased, and avoidance of abrupt withdrawal by tapering the dose gradually (Busto et al, 1986).

Buspirone (Buspar) is a new antianxiety agent distinct from the benzodiazepines. Studies suggest that it is as effective as benzodiazepines in the treatment of generalized anxiety disorder. There is no evidence suggesting it is an effective antipanic agent. Buspirone shows a consistently low incidence of sedation, psychomotor impairment, interaction with alcohol, dependency, and does not impair memory (Davis, 1985). There is preliminary information that buspirone does not cause ventilatory impairment. Buspirone does not block benzodiazepine withdrawal symptoms, creating a problem in switching over to buspirone. The major limitations of buspirone include efficacy in patients recently treated with benzodiazepines, the need for multiple doses and a lag period of 1 to 2 weeks for full anxiolygic effects to appear. These latter features limit patient acceptance (Davis, 1985)

Propranolol and Related Drugs

Anxiety is characterized by a number of autonomic symptoms such as palpitations, rapid heartbeat, tremor, tingling, cold sweats, chest tightness, etc. These symptoms could, in part, be caused by the secretion of epinephrine during stress. Many of the symptoms can be blocked by a beta adrenergic receptor blocker. Propranolol (Inderal), as well as other beta blockers, have been used for general anxiety and for anxiety provoking situations such as public speaking. Ongoing research has verified their usefulness in situational anxiety and less impressive results in panic disorders. These drugs are generally prescribed for a variety of medical conditions such as hypertension and angina pectoris. Their side effects include hypotension and depression. They are contraindicated in asthma and cardiac conditions for which slowing of the heart would be detrimental (Cole, Altesman, & Weingarten, 1979).

Sedative/Hypnotics

Drugs used to facilitate sleep are known as hypnotics. They are CNS depressants that, in large doses, can produce anesthesia and death. Most of the hypnotic agents effectively induce and maintain sleep the first few days, but this effect diminishes after several days. These agents should only be used for very brief periods because of the addiction and abuse potential. The side effects have already been discussed under the section on benzodiazepines and include hangover, memory impairment, and paradoxical combativeness.

Psychomotor Stimulants

Stimulants, which include amphetamine and methylphenidate, are of very limited clinical use in psychiatry. They are effective in treating hyperactive children (Chiarello & Cole, 1987). The main use of psychostimulants is the treatment of attention deficit disorder. Methylphenidate (Ritalin) and pemoline (Cylert) produce improved ability to concentrate and in classroom behavior in 75% to 90% of children. These drugs have potent central stimulant effects (Chiarello & Cole, 1987). They increase alertness and attention span in children, rather than a paradoxical tranquilizing effect as had once been thought. The short term use of methylphenidate in combination with tricyclic antidepressants in resistant depressions may also be justified (Davis, 1985). Methylphenidate has a place in the treatment of chronically depressed and medically ill patients, especially the elderly, whose conditions would not tolerate TCAs or MAOIs. Terminally ill cancer patients often can be helped with these agents to enjoy better quality during their final days. The effect of these agents are to improve mood, alertness, and to overcome the sedative effects of sedating pain killers. The improved energy can help these patients interact with their families. The use of psychostimulants in narcolepsy is controversial and TCAs often are more effective (Fish, 1970). The use of psychostimulants as a challenge test to predict antidepressant response has been advocated by some authors (Rickels, Gordon, Sansman, et al., 1970).

This involves administering a few test doses of these agents to aid in determining if an antidepressant might be used.

Because of side effects, the abuse potential and the easy development of psychic dependence, these drugs should be limited in use. Stimulant drugs can cause jitteriness, palpitations, insomnia, sexual dysfunction, and a severe rebound depression leading to addiction. Florid psychosis, resembling acute paranoid schizophrenia, can also be precipitated by these drugs (Chiarello & Cole, 1987). Anorexia is the most troublesome side effect and this can be reduced by giving the drug after meals. Children usually becomes tolerant to this side effect in the first couple of weeks of treatment. Mild transient insomnia, increased motor activity, abdominal pain, tearfulness, social withdrawal, and tachycardia are frequently encountered. The drug may lower the seizure threshold. Habituation to CNS stimulants has not been reported in children and there is no evidence suggesting that these drugs predispose to later addictive diseases (Chiarello & Cole, 1987).

Growth inhibition is reported. However, ultimate height and weight are not adversely affected, since growth rebound after discontinuance of the drug is proportional to growth suppression.

Antipsychotic Drugs

Psychoses are among the least understood and most devastating illnesses to affect mankind. Psychotic illnesses cause serious disruption in the lives of individuals and their loved ones and have a major impact on society by incapacitating significant numbers of people. The discovery of chlorpromazine (Thorazine) a scant 34 years ago was one of the significant advances in the understanding and treatment of psychotic illness. Since chlorpromazine became available in clinical practice, significant advances have been made in understanding the mechanisms and etiologies of psychosis. It is unlikely that a single cause will explain what appears to be a varied group of illnesses. Over 300,000 Americans alone are afflicted with schizophrenias, bipolar disorders, and other psychotic illnesses. Many others will develop transient psychotic conditions for a multitude of reasons. This section will discuss the drugs useful in treating these conditions.

To avoid confusion, these drugs are best referred to as antipsychotic drugs. The agents have also been called "neuroleptics" and "major tranquilizers." Unfortunately, all available therapeutic agents of this class produce some degree of extrapyramidal effects (EPS) (e.g., tremor, shuffling gait) that must be managed when these drugs are administered to patient. The connection between the beneficial effects and the side effects has become better understood as dopamine receptor blockage has been recognized as the most likely mechanism of antipsychotic drug action. There are now about 20 antipsychotic drugs on the market, divided among five distinct chemical classes.

Only eight or nine of these products have widespread clinical use by practitioners. These antipsychotic drugs appear to act by the mechanism of dopamine blockage, suggesting the possibility that in schizophrenia, the underlying disease mechanism may involve an abnormality of dopamine release or receptor sensitivity (Farde, 1989).

One experimental antipsychotic compound, clozapine, appears to exert its action in another way. This drug was released early in 1990 and could herald a new direction in the treatment of these disorders, and most of the current antipsychotics may become obsolete in the next 10 years (Meltzer, 1989).

The clinical use of antipsychotic drugs is primarily directed toward syndrome and symptoms. The main target symptoms are disturbed psychomotor behavior, abnormal affect, psychotic perceptual disturbances (hallucinations), delusional thinking, catatonic behavior, autistic withdrawal, and others (Schultz & Pata, 1989).

Most experts agree that the various agents do not differ in their antipsychotic effects if equivalent doses are given. Although there is little evidence that any of these drugs is clearly superior to another in antipsychotic effect, they do have different side effect profiles. Since specific side effects may be more or less problematic in particular patients, this is one basis for the choice of a particular drug. Although there are no clear indications for specific antipsychotic drugs, clinicians observe that patients who fail to respond to one antipsychotic drug may respond to another, even though it belongs to the same chemical group. As plasma levels of antipsychotics reveal, there are extreme individual variations in absorption, metabolism, and excretion of psychoactive drugs which may explain why a certain person may respond to one drug but not another (Kane, 1989). A basic pharmacotherapeutic requirement is that these drugs be given in a generally accepted dosage range and over a certain time. There is little to be gained in changing hastily from one drug to another without an adequate clinical trial.

Therapy with antipsychotic drugs can be divided into three phases. The initial phase of treatment is generally aimed at providing behavioral control and reducing agitation, fear, delusions, and hallucinations. This can take from hours to weeks (Kane, 1989).

The next phase of antipsychotic chemotherapy involves stabilization and gradual reduction of the medication dosage to receive the best possible control using the lowest possible dose, thereby reducing the patient's vulnerability to drug side effects.

The third phase of treatment of the psychotic patient may be referred to as maintenance therapy, and involves long term continuous administration of the lowest possible dose of effective medication to prevent recurrence of the illness. Clearly, a great deal of emotional support to patients and their families, rehabilitation services, and community networking are essential to

maximize the patient's recovery and reintegration. Specific psychotherapeutic intervention is beyond the scope of this chapter. It has been repeatedly
shown, however, that psychotherapeutic interventions in the absence of
adequate drug treatment of psychotic disorders lead to suboptimal outcomes.

In the schizophrenic patient, treatment is generally best accomplished by
starting and continuing treatment with a single antipsychotic agent, provided
the patient can tolerate this medication without incapacitating side effects. If
side effects do develop, they can usually be managed by dosage adjustment,
addition of an antiparkinsonism medication, or changing to a different
medication.

In the treatment of the acutely manic patient, treatment is usually initiated
with an antipsychotic drug in conjunction with lithium carbonate. Then the
antipsychotics can usually be withdrawn gradually and the patient maintained
on lithium.

Treatment of the psychotically depressed patient is usually initiated by
using antipsychotic drugs to manage the delusions, along with an antidepressant. The patient with psychosis should generally receive maintenance
medication consisting either of antidepressant drugs alone or in combination
with antipsychotic drugs or lithium. The duration for maintenance therapy
varies. About 70% of psychotically depressed patients who respond to
pharmacologic treatment are off all medication within 1 year. The majority of
schizophrenic patients may require maintenance medication for many years,
possibly for life.

Side Effects

The side effects of the antipsychotic drugs can be classified as follows:
autonomic effects, extrapyramidal effects, other central nervous system
effects, behavioral toxicity, allergic reactions, agranulocytosis, skin and eye
effects, and endocrine effects.

The autonomic side effects that can occur include dry mouth, blurred
vision, skin flushing, constipation, paralytic ileus, mental confusion, and
postural hypotension. Dry mouth is one of the most often complained about
side effect and can be managed by advising the patient to rinse the mouth
frequently with water. The use of sugarless chewing gum can be helpful.
Regular sugared gum and candy should be avoided since the sugar added to
the dry mouth can predispose to fungal infections and dental caries. Patients
usually develop tolerance to blurred vision, which is usually problematic only
in the first few weeks of treatment. The blurred vision can be managed with
reassurance that this is temporary and by the use of magnifying lenses.
Inexpensive premade glasses are readily available in drug stores at various
strengths of magnification.

Orthostatic hypotension may occur in the first few days of treatment. The main danger of this is that patients may fall and injure themselves. Instructing the patient to arise slowly from a lying to standing position is important. Support hose may help by preventing blood pooling in the lower extremities. The most dramatic and the most theoretically important group of side effects shown by all the antipsychotic drug agents are the extrapyramidal reactions (EPS) (Kane, 1989). These side effects are classified into three categories: parkinsonian syndrome, dystonias, and akathesia. The parkinsonian syndrome consists of a mask-like face, tremor at rest, rigidity, shuffling gait, and motor retardation (bradykinesia) (Kane, 1989). This syndrome is symptomatically identical to idiopathic parkinsonism (Parkinson's disease). The dystonias consist of a broad range of bizarre movements of the tongue, face, and neck. The patient may experience severe muscle spasms of the neck. The tongue may protrude and partially obstruct the airway. The patient's eyes may roll upward (oculogyric crisis). Akithesia is a motor restlessness in which the patient has a great urge to move about and may not be able to sit or stand still.

These side effects are fairly common, vary in intensity, and are easily reversible. They are very distressing to the patient and if not properly managed, can lead to medication noncompliance, thereby compromising the patient's chances for recovery.

Younger patients tend to experience dystonic reactions more often than middle-aged patients, possibly because they have higher levels of dopamine. The acute dystonias typically occur early in the course of treatment even with small doses of antipsychotic drugs. They usually resolve within minutes of intramuscular administration of one of the antiparkinsonisan drugs such as benztropine (Cogentin), diphenhydramine (Benedryl), or trihexphenidryl (Artane). Amantadine (Symmetrel) is helpful with parkinsonian symptoms and akithesia.

There is controversy in psychiatry about whether one should prophylactically administer an antiparkinsonian medication to all patients being treated with antipsychotic drugs or give it only if side effects occur. Common practice is to co-administer antiparkinsonian drugs and then attempt to discontinue them gradually after about 3 months.

A rare syndrome described as the neuroleptic malignant syndrome (NMS) characterized by muscular rigidity, hyperthermia, altered consciousness, and autonomic dysregulation has been recognized (Kane, 1989). This is a potentially fatal complication that must be diagnosed and treated early. Discontinuance of the drug, supportive measures such as lowering body temperature, using muscle relaxants such as dantrolene, IV fluids, and possibly, emergency electroconvulsive therapy, are life-saving. Antipsychotics can usually be safely restarted if needed when the crisis is over. There is little evidence implicating one class of antipsychotic drug over another. There may be a greater liklihood of NMS when multiple psychotropic drugs are used together.

Tardive dyskinesia (TD) is an extrapyramidal syndrome that emerges relatively late in the course of antipsychotic treatment. Long term, high dose treatment increases the incidence of TD. TD may also appear days or weeks after antipsychotics are discontinued. This syndrome is sometimes irreversible and no consistently effective treatment has been identified. TD presents with facial grimaces, bucco-lingual movements such as lip smacking, lateral jaw movements, flicking of the tongue, jerking movements of the arms (chorea), and athetoid movements of arms and fingers. Neck and trunk movements can also be found. Symptoms are absent during sleep. The overall incidence of TD is about 15% and is correlated with length of exposure to the drug and total lifetime dose (Glazer, 1989).

As with all forms of treatment, careful decisions have to be made concerning the risks of a drug versus its potential benefits. Psychosis is a frightening, debilitating affliction and usually renders patients dysfunctional. The antipsychotic drugs, despite their liabilities, have helped hundreds of thousands to live outside of psychiatric institutions, and in conjunction with psychotherapies, social and occupational rehabilitation, to lead relatively normal lives.

The various antipsychotic drugs and their side effects are shown in Table 11-6.

Table 11-6
Antipsychotic Drugs

Name			Side Effects of Antipsychotics	Name		
Class	Generic	Trade		Class	Generic	Trade
Aliphatic	Chlorpromazine	Thorazine	Dry mouth and throat	Piperidine	Thioridazine	Mellaril
	Trifluoproaine	Vesprin	Blurred vision Cutaneous flushing Constipation		Mescridazine	Berentil
					Piperacelazine	Quide
Piperazine	Prochlorperazine	Compazine	Urinary retension Paralytic ileus Mental confusion Miosis	Butyrophenones	Haloperidol	Haldol
	Perphenazine	Trilafon			Pimozide	Orap
	Trifluoperazine	Stelazine	Myariasis Orthostatic hypotension	Thioxanthines	Chlorprethizene	Taractan
	Fluphenazine	Prolixin			Thiothixene	Navane
		Permitil	Parkinsonian Syndrome: Tremor at rest Drooling Mask-like face Rigidity Shuffling Gait Motor Retardation			

Table 11-6 *continued*
Antipsychotic Drugs

Name				Name		
Class	Generic	Trade	Side Effects of Antipsychotics	Class	Generic	Trade
	Acetophenazine	Tindal	Dyskinesias: Tardive dyskinesia	Dibenzoxazepines	Loxapine	Loxitane
	Butaperazine	Repoise	Sedation	Dihydroindoline	Molindone	Moban
	Carphenazine	Proketazine	Bizarre dreams Uncoordination Confusion Dermatitis Photosensitivity Deposits in the cornea and lens Breast engorgement and lactation Weight gain Delayed ejaculation Jaundice Blood dyscrasias			

Lithium

Lithium has been extensively studied for a variety of clinical conditions. Its widest and best known application is in the treatment of mania and bipolar disorders. The main use of lithium today is for prophylaxis in recurrent affective disorders. It has been shown to be highly effective in preventing both depressive and manic episodes of affective disorder and schizoaffective disorders. The prophylactic effect does not differ in unipolar and bipolar patients. Lithium prevents, or at least reduces, intensity and duration of affective episodes in the majority of these patients. A patient with an atypical affective or cyclic psychosis responding to prophylactic lithium treatment should be maintained on it (Schou, 1989). Other indications, such as therapy for schizophrenia, alcoholism, and some types of personality disorders, are less clearly established (Ortiz, Dabbaugh, & Gershan, 1984). Its use as adjunctive therapy for depression is becoming more popular as is its use in treatment resistant migraine headaches, thyrotoxicosis, and premenstrual syndrome.

Because of its slower effect and lack of sedation, lithium alone often cannot adequately control acute manic symptoms. Therefore, lithium and antipsychotic drugs are often combined during acute phases of the disorder (Abou & Cooper, 1987).

Numerous trials have shown that the prophylactic effect of lithium in affective disorders is obtained in only 70% to 80% of cases. Because of this, along with the fact that a significant number of patients are lithium intolerant, other bipolar drugs are being tried, particularly the anticonvulsants carbamaz-epin (Tegretol) and sodium valproate (Depakote).

Lithium is contraindicated in patients with severe cardiovascular disease, in diseases in which dietary sodium is restricted, in Addison's disease, and the first 4 months of pregnancy. Women on lithium should be counseled against breast feeding. The use of lithium with diuretics is a relative contraindication since urinary sodium loss and volume depletion can produce toxic lithium blood levels. Lithium is relatively contraindicated in certain kidney diseases (Ortiz et al., 1984).

Side effects occurring in the initial period of lithium therapy tend to disappear with continued treatment. They include polydipsia (excessive thirst), polyuria (excessive urination), fine hand tremor, and diarrhea. Less often found are nausea, sedation, dizziness, fatigue, and abdominal discomfort. Side effects occurring days or weeks later include edema, weight gain, and myxedema (hypothyroidism). It is rarely necessary to discontinue lithium because of side effects.

Lithium produces a generally benign lowering in the concentration of circulatory thyroid hormones. In most cases the effects of lithium on thyroid function are not of sufficient magnitude to require treatment. If necessary, thyroid supplementation may be administered. Underlying thyroid disorder is not a contraindication to lithium therapy per se.

Lithium produces two distinct categories of renal effects. The most frequent and benign effect is a nephrogenic diabetes insipidus. The other, more serious effect, is damage to kidney morphology (structure) (Ortiz et al., 1984). Several contradictory studies raise doubt whether these lesions are due to lithium alone. With appropriate patient selection, careful renal evaluation, and close clinical and lab follow up, the risk of kidney disease is remote.

The effects of lithium on the central nervous system range from commonly observed mild effects to irreversible life threatening brain damage in rare instances of severe toxicity. The neurotoxic reaction is characterized by symptoms of organic brain syndrome such as disorientation, confusion, dysarthia (slurred speech), ataxia, reduced concentration, somnolence, leth-argy, and extrapyramidal signs (Ortiz et al., 1984). Although neurotoxicity has been reported with lithium alone, the extreme neurotoxic syndrome is more often associated with the combination of lithium and an antipsychotic drug (Abou & Cooper, 1987). This neuroleptic malignant syndrome may be caused by the antipsychotic drug itself, whether the addition of lithium causes a greater vulnerability is still not clear (Schou, 1989).

Prior to lithium therapy, a general medical workup should be done including physical examination, EKG, complete blood count, kidney function tests, urinalysis, and thyroid functions. Renal and thyroid functions should be rechecked at least once a year. Treatment is usually started at a dose expected to produce plasma levels within the therapeutic range. After 1 week of continued treatment with a constant dose, the blood level is checked and dosage is adjusted accordingly until effective serum levels of 0.5 to 0.8 mg/L are attained. In manic states, higher levels may be necessary. Once the lithium level is established it should be checked monthly the first half year and then every 3 months thereafter.

Lithium is available as lithium carbonate (Eskalith, Lithonate, Lithane) in capsules and liquid (as citrate). It is also available in sustained release form (Lithobid, Eskalith CR) in various doses (300 mg, 450 mg), and as lithium citrate, lithium acetate, and lithium sulphate. The sustained release forms may be preferable because they might avoid peaks in blood levels and are apt to cause fewer side effects. These medications are administered in divided doses, two or three times per day, although single doses may be as effective with fewer renal effects (Schou, 1989).

Calcium Channel Blockers

Calcium channel blockers (CCBs) are a recently introduced class of drugs with purported usefulness in the treatment of diverse psychiatric illnesses. At least three such drugs, verapamil, nifendipine and diltiazem are available in the US.

It has long been known that disturbances in extracellular calcium levels can produce a number of psychiatric problems. Extracellular calcium may influence disorder via effects on transmitter release. Calcium effects on pathophysiology of primary psychiatric disorders is likely intracellular (Hoschl, Blahos, & Kabes, 1986). Calcium entry into the cytoplasm activates a variety of enzymes, alters structural proteins, and is necessary for neurotransmitter release.

Several authors suggest a role for calcium channel blockers in the treatment of depression and mania reported dramatic decreases in the manic symptoms. The authors noted the absence of significant side effects and the ability to reduce more toxic antipsychotic drugs in many patients. Studies of the effectiveness of calcium channel blockers in schizophrenia are few and inconclusive but this is an intriguing area for further study.

Calcium channel blockers are labeled for treatment of cardiovascular disorders and are not yet FDA approved for psychiatric conditions. The major side effects include AV block, bradycardia (slowed heart rate), constipation, heartburn, nausea, flushing, and peripheral edema (Hoschl et al, 1986).

In conclusion, the calcium channel blockers are a class of agents with some treatment potential in psychiatry. They are generally safe and well-tolerated. Preliminary reports are interesting but the numbers of well controlled studies is small. More studies are necessary to follow up promising leads suggested by early reports of effectiveness in psychiatric syndromes.

General Considerations

Regardless of the diagnosis and the drug, there are some general considerations related to prescribing and monitoring psychopharmacological treatments. Depression will be discussed here as an example of clinical decision making about pharmacotherapy and as a way to introduce general considerations about psychotropic drug.

There is a growing body of information pertinent to treatment decisions concerning the efficacy of using drugs and psychotherapy in combination for the management of the acute depressive episode, and for long term treatment to prevent relapses and enhance the social and familial adjustment of patients. Decisions about medication should be made on the basis of specific diagnoses, availability of drug and non-drug treatments and evidence about their efficacy for particular kinds of individuals and situations.

There are some misconceptions that interfere with decision making. A commonly held view is that all patients should have psychotherapy. That view is still common throughout the practicing community as well as many parts of the public sector, particularly the better educated, middle class community who have come to accept a psychologically-oriented value system. However, in some situations, psychotherapy alone can be harmful. There are at least four groups of depressed patients that should receive medication in combination with some form of psychotherapy and for whom the evidence indicates that psychotherapy alone is ineffective and possibly harmful. These are psychotic or delusional depression; bipolar disorder; endogenous or melancholic symptom complex; and agoraphobia.

A second set of misconceptions is that all depressed patients should be medicated. Just as psychotherapists are at fault for their blanket prescription of psychotherapy, the advocates of biological psychiatry are potentially at fault for advocating that all forms of depression should be treated with medication. Particularly in the non-endogenous, non-psychotic, non-bipolar forms of depression, the patient can do equally well or better with some form of psychotherapy (Klerman, 1984).

In other words, there are popular misconceptions and professional biases both for and against drug treatment that can interfere with good treatment decisions.

As noted in a previous chapter, the distinction between endogenous and neurotic depression has been questioned. Sometimes the term neurotic depression is used to refer to depressions that arise as a consequence of character or personality maladjustments of the patient and, in that sense, are not precipitated by events, but arise because of the patient's long standing character conflicts. Sometimes it refers to depression that arises from a life event also called "reactive" or "situational" depression. Sometimes it refers to less severe depression. There is very good evidence that this type of depression responds to medication as well as to psychotherapy, alone or in combination. The decision to use medication should not be based on the presence or absence of precipitating life events but on the existing symptoms and their intensity. For the patient who has both the symptom complex and the adverse life event, as is the case in the majority of outpatients, the combination of drugs and psychotherapy is highly successful.

Similarly, medication may be useful for patients whose depressions are chronic or who have long term character problems. A high percentage of patients with character pathology present with affective symptoms, usually a mild to severe depression.

This example makes it clear that effective use of psychotropic medications requires an understanding of drug effects, the diagnosis and origins of the disorder, and the specific characteristics of the individual and his or her situation. Effective intervention requires careful decisions about medication, as well as coordination of pharmacological with other interventions. Team members can provide valuable information about drug effects, both positive and negative, and about areas of function that need to be addressed through other forms of intervention. The best treatment is that in which decisions about medication are made carefully for each indivudal in the context of a comprehensive treatment plan.

References

Abou, M.T. & Copper, A.J. (1987). Acute treatment, long-term management and prophylaxis of affective disorders. *Psychiatric Annals,17*(5), 301-308.

Bassuk, E. & Schoonover, S. (1977). *The Practitioner's Guide to Psychoactive Drugs.* New York: Plenum Books.

Busto, V., Sellers, E., Naranjo. C., et al., (1986). Withdrawal reactions after long term therapeutic use of benzodiazepines. *New England Journal of Medicine, 315,* 854-859.

Chiarello R.J. & Cole, J., (1987). The use of psychostimulants in general psychiatry, a recommendation. *Archives of General Psychiatry, 44,* 286-296.

Cole, J., Altesman, R., Weingarten, C., (1979). Beta-blocking drugs in psychiatry. *McLean Hospital Journal, 4,* 40.

Cooper, G. (1988). The safety of fluoxetine - An update. *British Journal of Psychiatry, 153* (suppl 3), 77-86.

Davis, J. (1985). Antipsychotic drugs. In H. Kaplan & B. Sadock (Eds.), *Comprehensive Textbook of Psychiatry IV.* Baltimore: Williams and Wilkins, pp. 1481-1537.

Fang, J.C., Hinrich, J.V., & Ghonheim, M.H. (1987). Diazepam and memory: Evidence for spared memory function. *Pharmocology and Biochemistry of Behavior, 28,* 347-352.

Farde, L., (1989). PET studies of patients treated with antipsychotic drugs. *Psychiatric Annals, 19* (10), 530-535.

File, S. & Pellow, S. (1987). Behavioral pharmacology of minor tranquilizers. *Pharmacology Therapy, 35,* 265-290.

Fish, B. (1970). Drug use in psychiatric disorders of children. *American Journal of Psychiatry, 124,* 31-36.

Glazer, W.H. (1989). An introduction to tardive dyskinesia. *Psychiatric Annals, 19*(6), 288.

Gold, M., Potash, A.C., Extein, I. (1984) Laboratory Testing and Psychopharmacology. In J.G. Bernstein (Ed)., *Clinical Psychopharmacology.* Boston: John Wright, PSG, Inc., pp. 31.

Hackett, T. & Cassem, N. (Eds.) (1978). *Massachusetts General Hospital Handbook of General Psychiatry.* St. Louis: C.V. Mosby.

Haskell, D., Cole, J., Schniebolk, S., et al, (1986). A survey of diazepam patients. *Psychopharmacology Bulletin, 22,* 434-438.

Hoschl, C., Blahos, J., & Kabes, J. (1986). The use of calcium channel blockers in psychiatry. In C.E. Shagoss, R.C. Josiasson, W.H. Bridger, et al, (Eds.), *Biological Psychiatry 1985.* New York: Elsevior Science Publishing, pp. 330-332.

Jefferson, J. (1989). Cardiovascular effects and toxicity of anxiolytics and antidepressants. *Journal of Clinical Psychiatry, 50,* 365-375.

Kalinowsky, L.B., Hippius, H., & Helmfried, E.K., (1982). *Biological Treatments in Psychiatry.* New York: Grune and Stratton, pp. 129.

Kane, J.M. (1989). The current status of neuroleptic therapy. *Journal of Clinical Psychiatry, 50,* 322-328.

Klerman, G. (1984) Introduction. In J.G. Bernstein (Ed.), *Clinical Psychopharmacology.* Boston: John Wright, PSG, Inc., pp. 4-5.

Linnoila, M., Erwin, C.W., Brende, A., et al, (1983). Psychomotor effects of diazepam in anxious patients and healthy volunteers. *Journal of Clinical Psychopharmacology, 3,* pp. 88-96.

Lydiard, R.B., Larai, M.T., Ballenger, J.C., et al, (1987). Emergence of depressive symptoms in patients receiving alprazolam for panic disorder. *American Journal of Psychiatry, 144,* 664-665.

Mahta, N. (1983). The chemistry of buproprion. *Journal of Clinical Psychiatry, 44* (5 sec 2), 56-59.

Meltzer, H., (1989). Clozapine: Clincial advantage and biologic mechanisms. In S.C. Schults & C.A. Tammingo (Eds.), *Schizophrenia: Scientific Process.* New York: Oxford University Press, pp. 333-340.

O'Boyle, C., Barry, H., Fox, E., et al, (1982). Benzodiazepine-induced event amnesia following a stressful surgical procedure. *Psychopharmacology,*

9, 244-247.

Ortiz, A., Dabbagh, M., & Gershon, S. (1984). Lithium clinical use, toxicology, and mode of action. In J.G. Bernstein (Ed.), *Clinical Psychopharmacology* 2nd ed. Boston: John Wright. PSG, Inc., pp. 111-134.

Par, C.M.B. (1987). Monoamine oxidase inhibitors in the treatment of affective disorders. *Psychiatric Annals, 17,* 309-311.

Rickels, K., Gordon, P., Sansman, D., et al. (1970). Pemoline and methylphenidate in mildly depressed outpatients. *Clinical Pharmacologic Therapy, 11,* 698-709.

Roose, S. & Glassman, A. (1989). Cardiovascular effects of tricyclic antidepressants in depressed patients with and without heart disease. *Journal of Clinical Psychiatry Monograph, 7*(2), 1-18.

Schou, M. (1989). Lithium prophylaxis: Myths and realities. *American Journal of Psychiatry, 146*(5), 573-576.

Schuckit, H. (1988). *Clinical Dialogues in Psychiatric Disorders: Mood Disorders, A Pharmacologic Approach.* New York: Science and Medicine.

Schultz, S.C., & Pata, C.N. (1989). Pharmacologic treatment of schizophrenia. *Psychiatric Annals, 19*(10), 288.

Shader, R.I. & Greenblatt. (1984). Benzodiasepine overuse-misuse. *Journal of Clinical Psychopharmacology, 4,* 123-124.

Smiley, A. (1987). Effects of minor tranquilizers and antidepressants on psychomotor performance. *Journal of Clinical Psychiatry, 48*(12 suppl), 22-28.

Sussman, N. & Chou, J. (1988). Current issues in benzodiazepine use for anxiety disorders. *Psychiatric Annals, 18*(3), 139-144.

Tesar, G.E. & Rosenbaum, J.F. (1986). Successful use of chlorazepam in patients with treatment resistant panic. *Journal of Nervous and Mental Disorders, 174,* 477-482.

Appendix A
DSM-III-R Classification:
Axes I and II Categories and Codes

All official DSM-III-R codes are included in ICD-9-CM. Codes followed by a * are used for more than one DSM-III-R diagnosis or subtype in order to maintain compatibility with ICD-9-CM.

Numbers in parentheses are page numbers

A long dash following a diagnostic term indicates the need for a fifth digit subtype or other qualifying term.

The term *specify* following the name of some diagnostic categories indicates to add in parentheses after the name of the disorder.

NOS = Not Otherwise Specified

The current severity of a disorder may be specified after the diagnosis as:

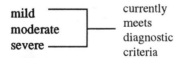

mild
moderate
severe

currently
meets
diagnostic
criteria

in partial remission
(or residual state)
in complete remission

DISORDERS USUALLY FIRST EVIDENT IN INFANCY, CHILD-HOOD, OR ADOLESCENCE

DEVELOPMENTAL DISORDERS
Note: These are coded on Axis II.

Mental Retardation (28)
317.00   Mild mental retardation
318.00   Moderate mental retardation
318.10   Severe mental retardation
318.20   Profound mental retardation
319.00   Unspecified mental retardation

Pervasive Developmental Disorders (33)
299.00   Autistic disorder (38)
                Specify if childhood onset
299.80   Pervasive developmental disorder NOS

Specific Developmental Disorders (39)
                Academic skills disorders
315.10   Developmental arithmetic disorder (41)
315.80   Developmental expressive writing disorder (42)
315.00   Developmental reading disorder (43)

Language and speech disorders
315.39   Developmental articulation disorder (44)
315.31* Developmental expressive language disorder (45)
315.31* Developmental receptive language disorder (47)

Motor skills disorder
315.40   Developmental coordination disorder (48)

315.90* Specific developmental disorder NOS

Other Developmental Disorders (49)
315.90* Developmental disorder NOS

Disruptive Behavior Disorders (49)
314.01   Attention-deficit hyperactivity disorder (50)

Conduct disorder, (53)
312.20   group type
312.00   solitary aggressive type
312.90   undifferentiated type
313.81   Oppositional defiant disorder (56)

Anxiety Disorders of Childhood or Adolescence (58)
309.21   Separation anxiety disorder (58)
313.21   Avoidant disorder of childhood or adolescence (61)
313.00   Overanxious disorder (63)

Eating Disorders (65)
307.10   Anorexia nervosa (65)
307.51   Bulimia nervosa (67)
307.52   Pica (69)
307.53   Rumination disorder of infancy (70)

307.50   Eating disorder NOS

Gender Identity Disorders (71)
302.60   Gender identity disorder of childhood (71)
302.50   Transsexualism (74)
             Specify sexual history: asexual, homosexual, heterosexual, unspecified

302.85* Gender identity disorder of adolescence or adulthood, non-transsexual type (76)
             Specify sexual history: asexual, homosexual, heterosexual, unspecified
302.85* Gender identity disorder NOS

Tic Disorders (78)
307.33   Tourette's disorder (79)
307.22   Chronic motor or vocal tic disorder (81)
307.21   Transient tic disorder (81)
             Specify: single episode or recurrent
307.20   Tic disorder NOS

Elimination Disorders (82)
307.70   Functional encopresis (82)
             Specify: primary or secondary type
307.60   Functional enuresis (84)
             Specify: primary or secondary type
             Specify: nocturnal only, diurnal only, nocturnal and diurnal

Speech disorders Not Elsewhere Classified (85)
307.00* Cluttering (85)
307.00* Stuttering (86)

Other Disorders of Infancy, Childhood, or Adolescence (88)
312.23   Elective mutism (88)

313.82 Identity disorder (89)
313.89 Reactive attachment disorder of infancy or early childhood (91)
307.30 Stereotypy/habit disorder (93)
314.00 Undifferentiated attention-deficit disorder (95)

ORGANIC MENTAL DISORDERS (97)

Dementias Arising in the Senium and Presenium (119)

Primary degenerative dementia of the Alzheimer type, senile onset, (119)
290.30 with delirium
290.20 with delusions
290.21 with depression
290.00* uncomplicated
(Note: code 331.00 Alzheimer's disease on Axis III)

Code in fifth digit:
1 = with delirium, 2 = with delusions,
3 = with depression, 0* = uncomplicated
290.1x Primary degenerative dementia of the Alzheimer type, presenile onset, _____ (119)
(Note: code 331.00 Alzheimer's disease on Axis III)
290.4x Multi-infarct dementia, _____ (121)

290.00* Senile dementia NOS
Specify etiology on Axis III if known (e.g., Pick's disease, Jakob-Creutzfeldt disease)

Psychoactive Substance-Induced Organic Mental Disorders (123)

Alcohol
303.00 intoxication (127)
291.40 idiosyncratic intoxication (128)

291.80 Uncomplicated alcohol withdrawal (129)
291.00 withdrawal delirium (131)
291.30 hallucinosis (131)
291.10 amnestic disorder (133)
291.20 Dementia associated with alcoholism (133)

Amphetamine or similarly acting sympathomimetic
305.70* intoxication (134)
292.00* with drawal (136)
292.81* delirium (136)
292.11* delusional disorder (137)

Caffeine
305.90* intoxication (138)

Cannabis
305.20* intoxication (138)
292.11* delusional disorder (140)

Cocaine
305.60* intoxication (141)
292.00* withdrawal (142)
292.81* delirium (143)
292.11* delusional disorder (143)

Hallucinogen
305.30* hallucinosis (144)
292.11* delusional disorder (146)
292.84* mood disorder (146)
292.89* Posthallucinogen perception disorder (147)

Inhalant
305.90* intoxication (148)

Nicotine
292.00* withdrawal (150)

Opioid
305.50* intoxication (151)
292.00* withdrawal (152)

Phencyclidine (PCP) or similarly acting arylcyclohexylamine

305.90*	intoxication (154)
292.81*	delirium (155)
292.11*	delusional disorder (156)
292.84*	mood disorder (156)
292.90*	organic mental disorder NOS

Sedative, hypnotic, or anxiolytic

305.40*	intoxication (158)
292.00*	Uncomplicated sedative, hypnotic, or anxiolytic withdrawal (159)
292.00*	withdrawl delirium (160)
292.83*	amnestic disorder (161)

Other or unspecified psychoactive substance (162)

305.90*	intoxication
292.00*	withdrawal
292.81*	delirium
292.82*	dementia
292.83*	amnestic disorder
292.11*	delusional disorder
292.12	hallucinosis
292.84*	mood disorder
292.89*	anxiety disorder
292.89*	personality disorder
292.90*	organic mental disorder NOS

Organic Mental Disorders associated with Axis III physical disorders or conditions, or whose etiology is unknown. (162)

293.00	Delirium (100)
294.10	Dementia (103)
294.00	Amnestic disorder (108)
293.81	Organic delusional disorder (109)
293.82	Organic hallucinosis (110)

293.83	Organic mood disorder (111)
294.80*	Organic anxiety disorder (113)
310.10	Organic personality disorder (114)

Specify if explosive type

294.80* Organic mental disorder NOS

PSYCHOACTIVE SUBSTANCE USE DISORDERS (165)

Alcohol (173)

303.90	dependence
305.00	abuse

Amphetamine or similarly acting sympathomimetic (175)

304.40	dependence
305.70*	abuse

Cocaine (177)

304.20	dependence
305.70*	abuse

Hallucinogen (179)

304.50*	dependence
305.30*	abuse

Inhalant (180)

304.60	dependence
305.90*	abuse

Nicotine (181)

305.10	dependence

Opioid (182)

304.00	dependence
305.50*	abuse

Phencyclidine (PCP) or similarly acting arylcyclohexylamine (183)

304.50*	dependence
305.90*	abuse

Sedative, hypnotic, or
anxiolytic (184)
304.10   dependence
305.40*   abuse

304.90* Polysubstance dependence
(185)
304.90* Psychoactive substance dependence NOS
305.90* Psychoactive substance abuse
NOS

SCHIZOPHRENIA (187)
Code in fifth digit: 1=subchronic, 2=
chronic, 3=subchronic with acute exacerbation, 4=chronic with acute exacerbation, 5=in remission, 0=unspecified.

Schizophrenia,
295.2x   catatonic, ——
295.1x   disorganized, ____
295.3x   paranoid, ____
Specify if stable type
295.9x   undifferentiated, ____
295.6x   residual, ____
Specify if late onset

DELUSIONAL (PARANOID) DISORDER (199)
297.10   Delusional (Paranoid) disorder
Specify type: erotomanic
grandiose
jealous
persecutory
somatic
unspecified

PSYCHOTIC DISORDERS NOT ELSEWHERE CLASSIFED (205)
298.80   Brief reactive psychosis (205)
295.40   Schizophreniform disorder
(207)
Specify: without good prognostic features or with good
prognostic features

295.70   Schizoaffective disorder (108)
Specify: bipolar type or
depressive type
297.30   Induced psychotic disorder
(210)
298.90   Psychotic disorder NOS
(Atypical psychosis) (211)

MOOD DISORDERS (213)
Code current state of Major depression
and Bipolar Disorder in fifth digit:
1 = mild
2 = moderate
3 = severe, without psychotic features
4 = with psychotic features (specify
mood-congruent or mood-incongruent)
5 = in partial remission
6 = in full remission
0 = unspecified

For major depressive episodes, specify
if chronic and specify in melancholic
type.

For Bipolar Disorder, Bipolar Disorder
NOS, Recurrent Major Depression, and
Depressive Disorder NOS, specify if
seasonal pattern.

Bipolar Disorders
Bipolar disorder, (225)
296.6x   mixed, ____
296.4x   manic, ____
296.5x   depressed, ____
301.13   Cyclothymia (226)
296.70   Bipolar disorder NOS

Depressive Disorders
Major Depression, (228)
296.2x   single episode, ____
296.3x   recurrent, ____
3004.40 Dysthymia (or Depressive
neurosis) (230)
Specify: primary or secondary type

Specify: Early or late onset

311.00 Depressive disorder NOS

ANXIETY DISORDERS (or Anxiety and Phobic Neuroses) (235)

Panic disorder (235)

300.21 with agoraphobia

Specify current severity of agoraphobic avoidance

Specify current severity of panic attacks

300.01 without agoraphobia

Specify current severity of panic attacks

300.22 Agoraphobia without history of panic disorder (240)

Specify with or without limited symptom attacks

300.23 Social phobia (241)

Specify if generalized type

300.29 Simple phobia (243)

300.30 Obsessive compulsive disorder (or Obsessive compulsive neurosis) (245)

309.89 Post-traumatic stress disorder (247)

Specify if delayed onset

300.02 Generalized anxiety disorder (251)

300.00 Anxiety disorder NOS

SOMATOFORM DISORDERS (255)

300.70* Body dysmorphic disorder (255)

300.11 Conversion disorder (or Hysterical neurosis, conversion type) (257)

Specify: single episode or recurrent

300.70* Hypochondriasis (or Hypochondriacal neurosis) (259)

300.81 Somatization disorder (261)

307.80 Somatoform pain disorder (264)

300.70* Undifferentiated somatoform

disorder (266)

300.70* Somatoform disorder NOS (267)

DISSOCIATIVE DISORDERS (or Hysterical Neuroses, Dissociative Type) (269)

300.14 Multiple personality disorder (269)

300.13 Psychogenic fugue (272)

300.12 Psychogenic amnesia (273)

300.60 Depersonalization disorder (or Depersonalization neurosis) (275)

SEXUAL DISORDERS (279)

Paraphilias (279)

302.40 Exhibitionism (282)

302.81 Fetishism (282)

302.89 Frotteurism (283)

302.20 Pedophilia (284)

Specify: same sex, opposite sex, same and opposite sex

Specify if limited to incest

Specify: exclusive type or nonexclusive type

302.83 Sexual masochism (286)

302.84 Sexual sadism (287)

302.30 Transvestic fetishism (288)

302.82 Voyeurism (289)

302.90* Paraphilia NOS (290)

Sexual Dysfunctions (290)

Specify: psychogenic only, or psychogenic and biogenic (Note: If biogenic only, code on Axis III)

Specify: lifelong or acquired

Specify: generalized or situational

Sexual desire disorders (293)

302.71 Hypoactive sexual desire disorder

302.79 Sexual aversion disorder

Sexual arousal disorders (294)
302.72*   Female sexual arousal disorder
302.72*   Male erectile disorder

Orgasm disorders (294)
302.73   inhibited female orgasm
302.74   Inhibited male orgasm
302.75   Premature ejaculation

Sexual pain disorders (295)
302.76   Dyspareunia
306.51   Vaginismus

302.70   Sexual dysfunction NOS

Other Sexual Disorders
302.90*   Sexual disorder NOS

SLEEP DISORDERS (297)
Dyssomnias (298)
Insomnia disorder
307.42*   related to another mental disorder (nonorganic) (300)
780.50*   related to known organic factor (300)
307.42*   Primary insomnia (301)
Hypersomnia disorder
307.44   related to another mental disorder (nonorganic) (303)
780.50*   related to a known organic factor (303)
780.54   Primary hypersomnia (305)
307.45   Sleep-wake schedule disorder (305)
    Specify: advanced or delayed phase type, disorganized type, frequently changing type
Other dyssomnias
307.40*   Dyssomnia NOS

Parasomnias (308)
307.47   Dream anxiety disorder (Nightmare disorder) (308)
307.46*   Sleep terror disorder (310)

307.46*   Sleepwalking disorder (311)
307.40*   Parasomnia NOS (313)

FACTITIOUS DISORDERS (315)
Factitious disorder
301.51   with physical symptoms (316)
300.16   with psychological symptoms (318)
3001.9   Factitious disorder NOS (320)

IMPULSE CONTROL DISORDERS NOT ELSEWHERE CLASSIFIED (321)
312.34   Intermittent explosive disorder (321)
312.32   Kleptomania (322)
31.31   Pathological gambling (324)
312.33   Pyromania (325)
312.39*   Trichotillomania (326)
31.39*   Impulse control disorder NOS (328)

ADJUSTMENT DISORDER (329)
Adjustment disorder
309.24   with anxious mood
309.00   with depressed mood
309.30   with disturbance of conduct
309.40   with mixed disturbance of emotions and conduct
309.28   with mixed emotional features
309.82   with physical complaints
309.83   with withdrawal
309.23   with work (or academic) inhibition
309.90   Adjustment disorder NOS

PSYCHOLOGICAL FACTORS AFFECTING PHYSICAL CONDITION (333)
316.00   Psychological factors affecting physcal condition
    Specify physical condition on Axis III

PERSONALITY DISORDERS
(335)
Note: These are coded on Axis II.
Cluster A
301.00   Paranoid (337)
301.20   Schizoid (339)
301.22   Schizotypal (340)
Cluster B
301.70   Antisocial (342)
301.83   Borderline (346)
301.50   Histrionic (348)
301.81   Narcissistic (349)
Cluster C
301.82   Avoidant (351)
301.60   Dependent (353)
301.40   Obsessive compulsive (354)
301.84   Passive aggressive (356)
301.90   Personality disorder NOS

V CODES FOR CONDITIONS NOT ATTRIBUTABLE TO A MENTAL DISORDER THAT ARE A FOCUS OF ATTENTION OR TREATMENT
(359)
V62.30   Academic problem
V71.01   Adult antisocial behavior

V40.00   Borderline intellectual functioning (Note: This is coded on Axis II.)

V71.02   Childhood or adolescent antisocial behavior
V65.20   Malingering
V61.10   Marital problem
V15.81   Noncompliance with medical treatment
V62.20   Occupational problem

V61.20   Parent-child problem
V62.81   Other interpersonal problem
V61.80   Other specified family circumstances
V62.89   Phase of life problem or other life circumstance problem
V62.82   Uncomplicated bereavement

ADDITIONAL CODES (363)
300.90   Unspecified mental disorder (nonpsychotic)
V71.09* No diagnosis or condition on Axis I
799.90* Diagnosis or condition deferred on Axis I

V71.09*   No diagnosis or condition on Axis II
799.90*   Diagnosis or condition deferred on Axis II

MULTIAXIAL SYSTEM
Axis I   Clinical Syndromes
          V Codes
Axis II   Developmental Disorders
          Personality Disorders
Axis III Physical Disorders and Conditions
Axis IV   Severity of Psychosocial Stressors
Axis V   Global Assessment of Functioning

Appendix B
Uniform Terminology Grid

PERFORMANCE AREAS

PERFORMANCE COMPONENTS	ACTIVITIES OF DAILY LIVING											WORK ACTIVITIES				PLAY OR LEISURE ACTIVITIES	
	Grooming	Oral Hygiene	Bathing	Toilet Hygiene	Dressing	Feeding and Eating	Medication Routine	Socialization	Functional Communication	Functional Mobility	Sexual Expression	Home Management	Care of Others	Educational Activities	Vocational Activities	Play or Leisure Exploration	Play Leisure Performance
A. SENSORIMOTOR COMPONENT																	
1. Sensory Integration																	
a. Sensory Awareness																	
b. Sensory Processing																	
(1) Tactile																	
(2) Proprioceptive																	
(3) Vestibular																	
(4) Visual																	
(5) Auditory																	
(6) Gustatory																	
(7) Olfactory																	
c. Perceptual Skills																	
(1) Stereognosis																	
(2) Kinesthesia																	
(3) Body-Scheme																	
(4) Right-Left Discrimination																	
(5) Form Constancy																	
(6) Position in Space																	
(7) Visual-Closure																	
(8) Figure Ground																	
(9) Depth Perception																	
(10) Topographical Orientation																	
2. Neuromuscular																	
a. Reflex																	
b. Range of Motion																	
c. Muscle Tone																	
d. Strength																	
e. Endurance																	
f. Postural Control																	
g. Soft Tissue Integrity																	

PERFORMANCE AREAS

PERFORMANCE COMPONENTS	Grooming	Oral Hygiene	Bathing	Toilet Hygiene	Dressing	Feeding and Eating	Medication Routine	Socialization	Functional Communication	Functional Mobility	Sexual Expression	Home Management	Care of Others	Educational Activities	Vocational Activities	Play or Leisure Exploration	Play Leisure Performance
ACTIVITIES OF DAILY LIVING												**ACTIVITIES**				**PLAY OR LEISURE ACTIVITIES**	
3. Motor																	
a. Activity Tolerance																	
b. Gross Motor Coordination																	
c. Crossing the Midline																	
d. Laterality																	
e. Bilateral Integration																	
f. Praxis																	
g. Fine Motor Coordination Dexterity																	
h. Visual-Motor Integration																	
i. Oral-Motor Control																	
B. COGNITIVE INTEGRATION AND COGNITIVE COMPONENTS																	
1. Level of Arousal																	
2. Orientation																	
3. Recognition																	
4. Attention Span																	
5. Memory																	
a. Short-term																	
b. Long-term																	
c. Remote																	
d. Recent																	
6. Sequencing																	
7. Categorization																	
8. Concept Formation																	
9. Intellectual Operations in Space																	
10. Problem Solving																	
11. Generalization of Learning																	
12. Integration of Learning																	
13. Synthesis of Learning																	

PERFORMANCE AREAS

PERFORMANCE COMPONENTS	ACTIVITIES OF DAILY LIVING											WORK ACTIVITIES				PLAY OR LEISURE ACTIVITIES	
	Grooming	Oral Hygiene	Bathing	Toilet Hygiene	Dressing	Feeding and Eating	Medication Routine	Socialization	Functional Communication	Functional Mobility	Sexual Expression	Home Management	Care of Others	Educational Activities	Vocational Activities	Play or Leisure Exploration	Play Leisure Performance
C. PSYCHOSOCIAL SKILLS AND PSYCHOLOGICAL COMPONENTS																	
1. Psychological																	
a. Roles																	
b. Values																	
c. Interests																	
d. Initiation of Activity																	
e. Termination of Activity																	
f. Self-Concept																	
2. Social																	
a. Social Conduct																	
b. Conversation																	
c. Self-Expression																	
3. Self-Management																	
a. Coping Skills																	
b. Time Management																	
c. Self-Control																	

Winnie Dunn, 1988. Reprinted with permission.

Glossary

Activities of daily living (ADL): The most basic self-care needs, including feeding, hygiene and grooming, toileting, and dressing.

Activity therapies: Therapies in which doing rather than talking is the primary mode of intervention.

Affect: "A pattern of observable behaviors that is the expression of a subjectively experienced feeling state (emotion)" (APA, 1987, p. 391). May be abnormally flat, labile, or inappropriate.

Agraphia: An inability to write, caused by impairment of CNS processing (i.e., not by paralysis).

Anhedonia: An inability to experience pleasure.

Aphasia: A communication deficit that may be expressive (i.e., the inability to effectively express a thought) or receptive (i.e., the inability to process what is being said). Occurs at the CNS level.

Ataxia: Poor balance and awkward movement, which results from CNS processing deficits.

Behaviorism: A theory of behavior and intervention that holds that behavior is learned; behaviors that are reinforced tend to recur, and those that are not to disappear.

Biofeedback: Provision of visual or auditory cues about physical processes (e.g., heart rate, muscle tension). May allow the individual to gain control of these processes.

Catatonia: Motor abnormality usually characterized by immobility or rigidity, in which no organic base has been identified.

Codependence: A condition in which substance dependence is subtly supported by the codependent who meets some need through the continued dependence on the individual.

Cognitive therapy: An approach to intervention that holds that emotional disturbance is the result of faulty belief systems.

Compulsion: Repetitive, purposeful behavior undertaken to diminish obsessive thoughts. Usually recognized as not genuinely helpful, but feels out of control to the individual.

Confabulation: Fabrication of facts that the individual cannot remember. The individual is not aware he/she is fabricating, thus is not intentionally lying.

Defense mechanisms: Patterns of thinking or behavior that are mediated at an unconscious level to provide psychic protection to an individual, e.g., projection, denial, etc.

Delusion: A fixed, firmly held belief system that is not in keeping with external reality.

Desensitization: A technique employed by behviorists to diminish fear and anxiety related to a stimulus, usually by pairing the stimulus with an incompatible response (e.g., relaxation).

Double depression: A diagnosis of major depressive episode superimposed on a diagnosis of dysthymia.

Educational approaches: Interventions that make use of factual learning/ teaching to change behaviors.

Ego: A concept developed by Freud, to describe that portion of the personality that mediates between wishes and conscience (superego).

Enuresis: Inability to control urine, usually bed-wetting.

Environmental approaches: Interventions based on changing the environment, e.g., changing support systems, modifying job, home, etc.

Extinction: A behavioral approach to discouraging a particular behavior by ignoring it and reinforcing other more acceptable behaviors.

Family therapy: Intervention with the entire family, based on the theory that individual psychological difficulties are symptomatic of family disorder.

Flight of ideas: Rapid continuous speech with rapid, unclear shifts from subject to subject.

Flooding: A behavioral technique in which the individual is inundated with an unpleasant stimulus on the theory that this will overwhelm and exhaust any anxiety response.

Group therapy: Any intervention directed toward groups of individuals rather than an individual alone.

Habilitation: Enabling for the first time, as in the case of someone who never acquired a particular skill, such as in mental retardation.

Hallucination: A sensory experience that does not match external reality.

Hyperactivity: Extreme activity, distractibility.

Instrumental activities of daily living (IADL): Self-care activities that are higher order than ADL; includes cooking, shopping, budgeting, home repair, etc.

Loose associations: Thoughts shift with little or no apparent logic.

Mainstreaming: The idea that individuals should, as much as possible, be in the least restrictive environment. Most often applies to educational settings, and having retarded children and others with dysfunction be placed in regular classrooms where possible.

Neurotic: An analytic concept that reflects psychodynamic conflicts that cause an individual difficulty. The individual remains in contact with reality.

Neurotransmitters: Chemical substances that convey nerve impulses at the synapses (gaps between nerve cells).

Obsession: An irresistible thought pattern, usually anxiety provoking, which intrudes on normal thought processes.

Panic attack: A state of extreme anxiety, usually including sweating, shortness of breath, chest pains, and fear. May come on unpredictably or as a result of a particular stimulus.

Paranoia: A thought pattern that reflects a belief that others are persecuting or attempting to harm one, in the absence of a realistic basis for such fears.

Perseveration: An inability to shift from thought to thought; persistence of an idea even when the subject changes.

Phobia: Fear of a particular stimulus, e.g., heights, snakes. The stimulus provokes both anxiety and avoidance of the stimulus.

Polydrug abuse: Abuse of several psychoactive drugs (e.g., alcohol and cocaine).

Prodromal: A preliminary phase of an illness that warns of upcoming major/primary symptoms.

Psychoanalysis: A verbal therapy based on analytic theories of intrapsychic conflict.

Psychodynamic: Any therapy that examines intrapsychic conflicts.

Psychotic: A psychological state characterized by hallucinations and delusion, i.e., a loss of contact with reality.

Psychotropic medications: Drugs that act to relieve psychological symptoms.

Rational emotional therapy: A form of cognitive therapy. Intervention is designed to provide clients with cognitive understanding and control of emotions.

Reality orientation: A therapeutic intervention often used with demented patients. Includes both group techniques to remind the patient of facts, and patterned environment that provides memory cues.

Reality therapy: A form of therapy designed to provide individual with experience of reasonable consequences of actions.

Rehabilitation: Helping individuals regain skills and abilities that have been lost as a result of illness or disorder.

Reinforcement: A desired outcome of behavior. In behavior therapy, reinforcement is provided to encourage specific activities.

Relaxation: A technique that increases relaxation, including biofeedback, systematic relaxation exercises.

Reliability: The predictability of an outcome, regardless of observer. In diagnosis refers to the probability that several therapists will apply the same label to a given individual.

Self-concept: The view one has of oneself.

Self-esteem: The value one places on the attributes that comprise one's self-concept.

Self-help: Various methods by which individuals attempt to remedy their difficulties without making use of formal care providers. Examples include Alcoholics Anonymous and several organizations of former mental patients.

Sensory stimulation: A therapeutic intervention that uses patterned sensory input.

Sensory-integration: The ability of the CNS to process sensory information, also refers to a therapeutic intervention that uses strong kinesthetic and proprioceptive stimulation to attempt to better organize the CNS.

Sensory-motor: Therapeutic interventions that use both motor and sensory input in an effort to better organize the CNS.

Sheltered living: Living arrangements, such as group homes, that provide structure and supervision for individuals who do not require institutionalization but are not fully capable of independent living.

Social skills training: A cognitive/behavioral approach to teaching skills basic to social interaction.

Standard error: The possible range in which a person's "true" score on a test might fall; a number that recognizes the amount by which a score might vary on different days or in different situations.

Superego: An analytic concept that equates roughly to the conscience.

Systematic desensitization: A behavioral procedure that uses relaxation paired with an anxiety provoking stimulus in an attempt to reduce the anxiety response.

Therapeutic community: A structured inpatient environment that is designed to provide rehabilitative experience.

Thought form: The pattern or flow of ideas, the way in which thoughts take form.

Token economy: A structured inpatient environment in which behavioral principles are employed. Some form of token is used for reinforcement/ reward of desired behaviors.

Verbal therapies: Any therapy in which talk/discussion is the primary mode of intervention.

Waxy rigidity: A symptom of catatonia in which an individual will assume any position in which he/she is placed, and remain there until moved again.

Index